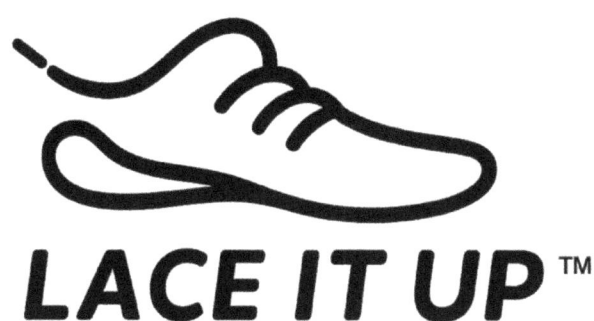

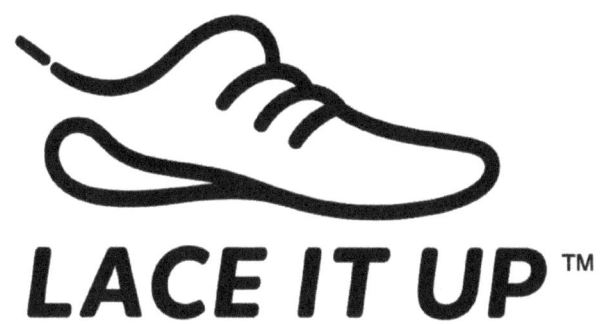

Eight Principles for Success in Team Sports

Gabriel Crespo

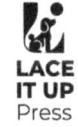

LACE IT UP Press

LACE IT UP: Eight Principles for Success in Team Sports
Copyright © 2025 by Gabriel Crespo.

All rights reserved.

No part of this publication may be reproduced or transmitted in any form or by any means, electronic or mechanical, including photocopying, recording, or any information storage and retrieval system, without permission in writing from the publisher, except for brief quotations in reviews or scholarly works.

Disclaimer: The information in this book is provided for educational purposes only and does not replace guidance from qualified coaches, athletic trainers, nutrition professionals, or healthcare providers. Readers assume all responsibility for their participation in any activity described.

Published by LACE IT UP Press
8735 Dunwoody Place #11248
Atlanta, GA 30350
ISBN (hardcover): 979-8-9933403-3-3

First edition
Printed in the United States of America

10 9 8 7 6 5 4 3 2 1

For Jackson and Carson

Who inspire me every day to lead, learn, and laugh. You are the reason I lace it up.

Contents

Introduction 1

Principle 1: Leadership.. 9

    What Leadership Looks Like 10

    Story: Dwyane Wade's Big Moment 11

    Story: Carson In Destin... 11

    Why Leadership Matters 12

    Different Leadership Styles 13

    Coaching vs. Leading.. 14

    Leading By Example 15

    The Three Everyday Qualities................................ 16

    Story: Running In the Rain 17

    Leaders Set Goals.. 19

    Leaders Make Decisions... 20

    Leadership: Key Takeaways.................................... 21

    Leadership: Reflections 22

    Leadership: Practice 23

Principle 2: Attitude 27

    Story: Jackson and the Power of a Positive Attitude 28

    Why Attitude Matters 30

    Mindset: The Engine of Attitude........................... 30

    Courage: The Muscle Inside Attitude 33

    Developing A Winning Attitude............................ 35

    The Bad Attitude Trap 36

    How to Handle Bad Attitudes................................ 38

    Analogy: The Mirror Effect................................... 38

    Story: The Toxic Parent 39

    Story: The Two Dogs Inside Us 40

    Attitude: Key Takeaways.. 42

Attitude: Reflections 42
Attitude: Practice 43

Principle 3: Communication 47
Story: Carson Finds His Voice 49
Story: Megan Rapinoe's Voice... 50
Why Communication Matters 51
Analogy: The Online Game Squad... 51
Active Listening: The Secret Weapon 52
Story: The Over-Eager Sideline Parent.................................... 53
Giving and Receiving Feedback... 55
Resolving Conflicts 56
Encouraging Unity and Inclusion.. 57
Story: The Silent Game 58
Communication: Key Takeaways... 60
Communication: Reflections 60
Communication: Practice 61

Principle 4: Effort... 65
What Effort Looks Like.. 66
Story: Jackson's Rising Stars Tournament............................... 67
Story: Michael Jordan's "Flu Game"....................................... 68
Bridging the Stories 69
Why Effort Matters.. 69
The Effort Spectrum 70
Story: The Team Manager Who Refused to Do the Minimum 71
Analogy: The Gas Tank.. 72
Story: The Empty Bleachers 73
Effort: Key Takeaways 74
Effort: Reflections 74

Effort: Practice 75

Principle 5: Intensity 79
    What Intensity Looks Like 80
    Analogy: The Light Bulb vs. the Laser 81
    Story: Allen Iverson's Practice 82
    Story: Kobe Bryant's Relentless Intensity 82
    Story: Coach Charles on 11 83
    Why Intensity Matters 85
    Analogy: The Volume Knob 85
    Intensity: Key Takeaways 86
    Intensity: Reflections 86
    Intensity: Practice 87

Principle 6: Teamwork 91
    What Teamwork Looks Like 92
    Analogy: The Puzzle 93
    Story: The Greatest Super Bowl Comeback 94
    Story: Carson the 5-Star Teammate 95
    Analogy: The Chain 97
    Why Teamwork Matters 98
    Teamwork: Key Takeaways 98
    Teamwork: Reflections 99
    Teamwork: Practice 99

Principle 7: Understanding 103
    What Understanding Looks Like 106
    Story: Jackson and the Seven-Touch Challenge 107
    Story: Derek Jeter's Flip and the Power of Preparation ... 108
    Understanding Yourself 109
    "I hate writing" options 113
    Understanding Others 116

    Understanding the Game 118
    Applying Understanding in Leadership 119
    Translating Understanding Beyond Sports 120
    Why Understanding Matters 121
    Understanding: Key Takeaways 121
    Understanding: Reflections 122
    Understanding: Practice 123
    21 Day Understanding Challenge 123

Principle 8: Practice 127
    What Practice Looks Like 128
    Story: Stephen Curry's Quiet Reps 129
    Story: The Wiffle Ball Reactor Drill 130
    Why Practice Matters 130
    The Practice Recipe 131
    Common Practice Traps (and quick fixes) 133
    Analogy: The Pencil 134
    Practice with Patience 134
    Practice With People 135
    Practice When You Are Not 100 Percent 136
    Tie It Back to Your Journal 137
    Practice: Key Takeaways 138
    Practice: Reflections 138
    Practice: Practice 139

Wrap: Tie It Up 143
    A new journey starts today 143
    What matters most going forward 144
    The 'Pass It On' Challenge 145
    Your next week, simple and clear 146
    Thank your people 146

A Final Word for Young Athletes 147
Final Word for Parents and Coaches 149
Acknowledgements 155
Appendix & Resources 159
Stay Connected with Team LACE IT UP..........................159
About the Author... 161
Notes 163

Introduction

Before every game, there is a small moment that changes everything. You bend down. You lace up. The noise fades. Your mind gets quiet. Your hands do something simple and steady while your body gets ready to do something hard.

That is what this book is about. Simple things that prepare you for hard things. Habits that hold when pressure hits. Choices you can control when the scoreboard feels like it controls you.

LACE IT UP is a playbook for youth athletes who want to grow on the field and off it. The letters stand for Leadership, Attitude, Communication, Effort, Intensity, Teamwork, Understanding, and Practice. Eight principles. Real stories. Clear tools. Nothing fluffy.

Why listen to me? I am not a famous pro. I am a dad, a husband, a working professional who leads teams for a living, and a coach at my core. I grew up in the Bronx, New York, where trouble was easy to find and good guidance mattered. After a rough run-in at 11, my mom signed me up for martial arts. That decision gave me structure, confidence, and a path. In the late 90s I moved to the Southeast. Now I spend a lot of time on the soccer fields with my boys, learning, cheering, and teaching. I have seen these principles work in my house, on my teams, and in my career.

Here is what this book will do. It will give you a clear standard to aim for. It will show you what good looks like with stories you can see yourself in. It will give you simple drills, questions, and habits that move you forward one day at a time.

Here is what this book will not do. It will not promise scholarships. It will not pretend you can skip the work. It will not offer you a magic pill or easy button. It will not tell you that talent is enough. It never is.

Let's make something clear right up front: This book is not going to teach you how to curve a soccer ball into the top corner, launch a home run over the fence, throw the perfect spiral, or drain free throws like a machine. That is not what it was designed for—and honestly, you should be glad. For specific skills, I defer you to the coaches, trainers, and experts who have spent years perfecting the drills and techniques that help athletes succeed in their chosen sports. They are the masters for the "how" of your sport, and you should soak up every tip and rep they offer.

This book's job is to give you everything you need on the mental, emotional, and team side—the invisible skills and rock-solid habits that separate the good from the great, in sports and in life after sports. Want to learn how to get tougher under pressure, work with absolutely anyone, show up on your worst day, or bounce back from a setback? That's what these pages are built for.

How to use this playbook

1. Read a principle. Take your time. Let the stories and lessons sink in.
2. Do the Reflections. Be honest. No one else has to see your answers.
3. Do the Practice. Small, specific actions beat big, vague goals.
4. Keep a Success Journal. Two to five minutes a day. Wins, challenges, one micro-goal, Energy Stars, one line with the word "yet." The greats write. You can too.
5. Bring it to your team. Share a drill. Share a phrase. Lift someone up.

Introduction

You will hear my voice in these pages. Dad. Mentor. Coach. New Yorker at heart. Southern by zip code. I believe in holding a high bar, keeping a warm tone and maintaining a casual demeanor. I believe nothing good is easy and nothing easy is good. I believe in laughing when the moment calls for it and locking in when it is time to work. You will get both here.

A quick story to set the tone. When my sons started club soccer, we were brand new to the sport. I knew enough to know that strikers score and goalkeepers live a tough life. For goalkeepers, people remember the shots you did not stop more than the saves you made. One day the coach asked who was brave enough to play keeper. My son Carson raised his hand. My stomach dropped. He struggled at first. He learned. He found his voice. He kept showing up and eventually became one of the best in his age group. That is the spirit of this book. Not perfect. Present. Not loud. Clear. Not flashy. Consistent.

Who is this for? The first jersey. The last tryout. The kid who plays a few minutes. The kid who starts every game. The parent who wants a better way to help. The coach who wants language the whole team can use. If you care about effort, respect, and growth, you are in the right place.

This book isn't just for athletes in huddles or locker rooms. Sure, soccer, basketball, baseball, and football teams are more likely to live these principles every day. But the heart of a team reaches far beyond those lines. If you're a tennis player, your coach and your training partners are your team. If you're a golfer, you have your caddie, your coach, your support crew. Boxers and MMA athletes might fight alone, but behind the ropes and octagons, there's a team of trainers, sparring partners, cut men, each one shaping the outcome. Even in individual sports, greatness is rarely a solo act.

Look closer, and you'll see that nobody goes on this journey alone. Everyone has a "team," whether it's family cheering from the stands, a mentor who sets the standard, or a friend who keeps you accountable. Champions build their tribe and lean on it when they need courage, direction, or truth. The principles in these pages—leadership, attitude, communication, effort, intensity, teamwork, understanding, and practice, aren't tied to the size of your roster. They work for anyone hungry to grow and willing to lift someone else along the way. As you read, think about who's in your corner and how you can be in theirs. That's where the real win starts.

What I ask from you:

1. Show up curious. Be a lifelong learner. Ask why. Take notes. Try new things.
2. Respect people. Parents, coaches, refs, teammates, opponents. Always.
3. Do the work. In games, in practice, in your journal, and in how you treat others.
4. Own your choices. Wins and losses teach. Effort and attitude are yours.

You will find humor in these pages. You will also find push. Some sections will feel easy to understand. Others will feel more challenging like sprints at the end of practice. That is good. Growth often shows up right after you want to stop. Get uncomfortable, and embrace the discomfort.

By the time you finish, you will know how to lead without a captain's band, how to build a winning attitude and bounce back on tough days, how to communicate with clarity, how to pair effort with intensity, how to be a five-star teammate, how to understand yourself and the game, and how to practice with purpose.

If you want a place to track habits, reflections, gratitude, and micro-goals as you read this book, I created two companion journals designed specifically for young athletes — the

Introduction

LACE IT UP Success Journal: Pre-Teen Edition and the LACE IT UP Success Journal: Teen Edition. They're optional, but they're a powerful tool to help athletes put these principles into action every day.

Laces in hand. Heart steady. Mind clear. Let us lace it up together and start with the first principle: Leadership.

"*Nothing Good is Easy and Nothing Easy is Good.*"

– Gabriel Crespo

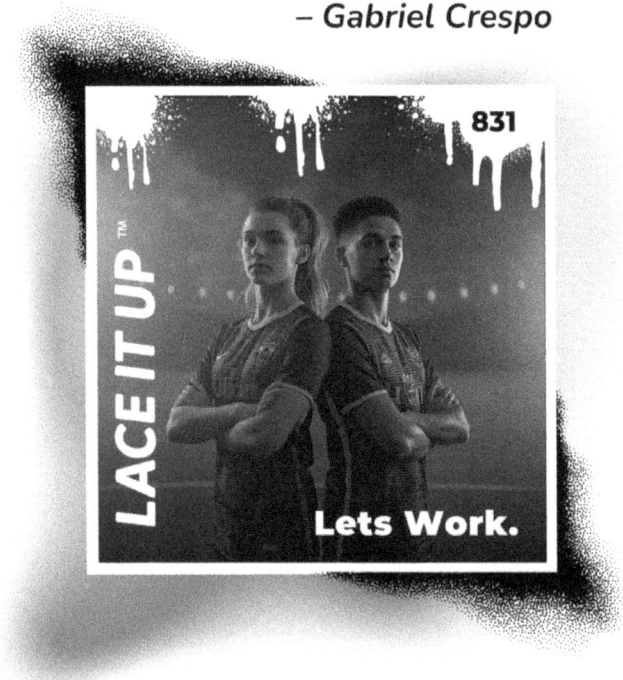

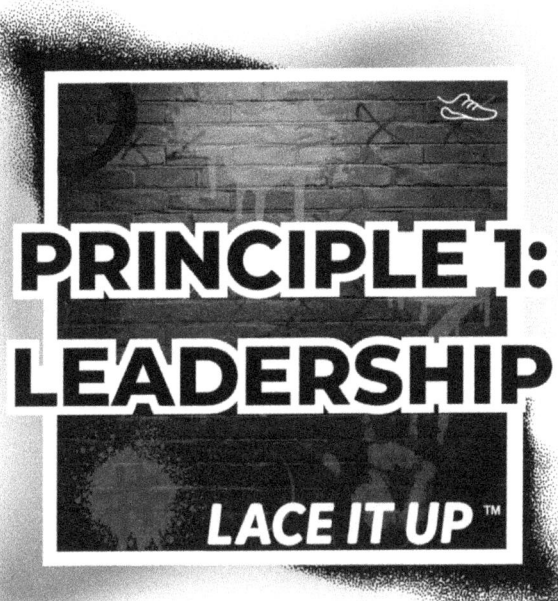

"Leaders aren't born, they are made. And they are made just like anything else, through hard work.."

– Vince Lombardi

Principle 1: Leadership

Before a single play is called and before any strategy takes shape, something deeper defines a team's journey—leadership. It isn't about the jersey you wear, the stats you post, or the cheers you earn. Leadership is built in the unseen moments, when nobody is watching and everything feels like an uphill battle. At its core, leadership pushes teams to reach beyond what's comfortable. It's not reserved for captains or coaches. It's a mindset, an attitude, a commitment, and a standard you choose to live by.

On every team, there's a turning point. It could be a huddle in the locker room, an extra sprint in practice, a word of encouragement after a tough loss. These moments, big and small, are where leaders show up. True leaders aren't louder or more decorated; they're the heartbeat of every practice, every challenge, every success. As athletes, the edge we find isn't just in skill, but in how we lift each other, how we hold ourselves accountable, and how we make those around us better.

The path to lasting victory starts when somebody decides to lead, and sometimes that's you. No age, no position, no spotlight required. Seriously. I've seen leaders of all ages emerge regardless of experience.

Let's break down what real leadership looks like, how it grows, and how every athlete, regardless of their role, can become the kind of leader whose legacy outlasts every scoreboard.

LACE IT UP

What Leadership Looks Like

Leadership is not a title or a speech. It is a pattern people can trust. It shows up when you enter a huddle, when you jog off at halftime and pull teammates with you, when you pick up cones and gather balls without being asked, when you line up the team's bags along the back of the bench. It is how you act after a turnover, how you carry yourself on the bench, and how you treat refs when a call goes against you.

Think about pressure moments. When the game gets chippy. A teammate is frustrated. The score is not in your favor. Some players read the room; others set it. Leaders set it. They choose calm over chaos, effort over excuses, and standards over shortcuts.

Ask yourself two questions: Are you a thermometer that only reflects the mood of the team, or a thermostat that sets it? If the sound was off and your teammates could only watch you, would they still know you are a leader? That is the test.

Signs of a leader:

1. Picks teammates up when they are down.
2. Works hard when no one is watching.
3. Shows respect to refs, coaches, teammates, and opponents.
4. Stays calm in tough moments.
5. Owns mistakes and fixes them.

Lesson: Leadership is not about who talks the loudest. You don't need to yell to lead. You need to show the standard. I call it modeling the way.

Principle 1: Leadership

Story: Dwyane Wade's Big Moment

Have you ever watched a player completely take over a game, almost like he decided, "We're not losing today"? That's what Dwyane Wade did in 2006. In the NBA Finals, his Miami Heat were down late in Game 3. The momentum was gone. Fans thought it was over.

But Wade refused to fold. He attacked the basket. He talked to his teammates with confidence. He played like the game still belonged to them. The Heat rallied, turned the game around, and went on to win the championship. Wade was named Finals MVP.

Lesson: A leader brings belief when everyone else is ready to doubt.

Story: Carson In Destin

Every now and then, sports delivers a memory that never leaves you. For me, it was a hot day on a field in Destin, Florida, surrounded by palm trees, sweaty parents clutching folding chairs, and a team of underdogs clutching hope like a lucky penny.

Carson was 9. His team was younger, smaller, and walked into a tournament with more nerves than swagger. They were facing kids 2 years older. From the start, they were fighting uphill. But what they lacked in experience, they made up for in guts and togetherness.

The final game went to penalty kicks. You could feel the tension in the air, parents frozen, coaches pacing, players shifting from one cleat to the other. All eyes on the kid in goal: my son. The game tied, it all came down to this moment. The other team's best shooter put the ball on the spot. Carson looked at his teammates, half nerves, half grin, chest out like a little lion. He thumped his chest, pointed to the squad, and yelled, "I got you!"

The shooter charged, unleashed a shot, and time seemed to slow. Carson dove, stretching every inch, and made the save, glove and ball, hope and belief colliding. Pure electricity. The sideline erupted like our country just won the World Cup. The team sprinted at Carson, mobbing him in a dogpile of sweaty hugs and wild shouts. We showered the team with splashes of water as the pros would do with champagne after winning a championship.

But here's what everyone missed if they only watched that save: leadership was building long before the whistle. All game, Carson was the steady flame, shouting encouragement after every shot, rallying teammates after every mistake, and telling every defender, "We got this, next play." He was the one who kept spirits high, even when their legs felt heavy or the scoreboard wasn't friendly.

Winning wasn't about one save. The real win was how he made others feel, how he lifted them, kept them steady, and turned a nervous bunch of kids into believers. That's leadership. That's impact. And that's a lesson you can take anywhere: Lead by how you show up for the people around you, especially when the moment gets big.

Championships, medals, and trophies are great, but what matters most is how you steady the ship. That day in Destin, Carson didn't just win a game. He showed his team, and every parent in the stands, what it means to lead with heart, humility, intention and real courage.

Why Leadership Matters

Plays win moments. Leadership wins seasons. It's the steady hand when the game turns for the worse, the voice that cuts through noise, and the example that reminds everyone what the standard is. When pressure hits, every team either locks in or falls apart.

Picture the hard parts. A bad call, a starter goes down, a mistake is made. Leaders lean-in to those moments. They settle the huddle, reset the plan, give direction, and make it safe for teammates to be honest. They turn frustration into focus and confusion into clarity.

Leadership also amplifies coaching. A coach can set a standard, but leaders carry it into every rep, every water break, every group text. They make the right habits contagious. They make the room lighter when it could get heavy. They keep the effort high even when the scoreboard says different.

Benefits of strong leadership for a team:

1. Teams stay connected when pressure hits.
2. Players work harder because effort becomes the standard.
3. Communication gets clear and honest.
4. Conflicts get handled instead of hidden.
5. Decisions get made with confidence.
6. Everyone is accountable.
7. Teams adjust to challenges instead of breaking.
8. Without leadership, talent gets wasted. With leadership, average teams overperform.

Different Leadership Styles

There is no single "right" way to lead. Different teams, moments, and personalities call for different approaches. The same leader who fires up a comeback on Saturday might spend Monday nights practice listening, sorting tension, and setting a clear plan. Think of leadership like a tool belt: you don't use a hammer for every job. You pick the tool that fits the moment, the person, and the goal.

LACE IT UP

Leadership experts have written about these approaches for decades. James MacGregor Burns first described transformational leadership in the 1970s[1], while Robert Greenleaf's work shaped the idea of servant leadership[2]. Others, like transactional and democratic leadership, come from well-established traditions in organizational psychology.

Transformational Leaders
- ✓ They inspire. They lift everyone's game and attitude.

Transactional Leaders
- ✓ The set clear goals and rewards. You do the work; you earn the result.

Servant Leaders
- ✓ They support the team first. They make people feel seen and valued.

Democratic Leaders
- ✓ They invite ideas. They listen before they decide.

Pro Tip: You should use more than one style. Great leaders adjust to what the team needs.

Coaching vs. Leading

Coaching and leading are not the same job. A coach can design a solid practice, run good drills, and teach technique, but still struggle to inspire or build a strong team culture. Some coaches get so caught up chasing wins that they forget to set the standard and model the way. Others mean well but never quite build trust. And many are simply human—new to the role, overwhelmed by other responsibilities, or balancing a lot on their plate. Coaches get my full empathy and should have yours too.

That's why I remind my boys: respect the coach, and lead as a teammate. Coaches can't see every play, feel every shift in energy, or know what happens when their back is turned. That's where player leadership comes in. Step up. Notice the little things. Encourage the kid who's frustrated, refocus the team when effort dips, and carry the standard when no one is watching.

Lesson: Great teams are built when players lead alongside their coaches.

Quick test I give my boys:

1. Do your teammates play harder when you are on the field?
2. Do they listen when you speak?
3. Do they mirror your effort?

Lesson: If the answers to the questions above are yes, you are leading.

Leading By Example

Every team has that one teammate, the one who never cheats a sprint, never skips a drill, and makes everyone around them want to work harder just by how they carry themselves. Can you picture someone like that? Is it you? If not, why not? That's leadership in its purest form.

When I was a kid, growing up a Yankees fan, Derek Jeter was that guy for me. He hustled on every play and owned his mistakes, no excuses. They didn't call him "The Captain" because of his stats, they called him that because of the standard he set every single day. Actions speak way louder than words.

Now, as I type this, I'm not at my desk or in a cozy writing nook. I'm actually sitting in my car, waiting for my son Jackson to wrap another late practice. Why? Because Jackson takes it on himself to stay late, help the coach gather cones, balls, pinnies, training tools, and load every last bit of gear into the coach's cart then into his truck. He's almost always the last one to leave the field. Sure, I'd love to be home by now getting dinner started. But I can't help but be proud that he's picked up this kind of leadership by example, the same kind that inspires everyone else to raise their game, too.

Great leaders show their teammates how to behave by what they do every single day. They work hard, arrive early, and stay late. They respect referees, coaches, teammates, and opponents. They stay positive, even when things get tough. Most importantly, they own their mistakes instead of making excuses, on the field and off.

Lesson: Minimize excuses, maximize effort.

The Three Everyday Qualities

I believe every great leader has three superpowers. No, not the kind you see in the movies. These don't come with capes, masks, or tight pants. They come from everyday choices: discipline, commitment, and work ethic.

1. **Discipline.** Follow your plan. Ignore distractions. Do the boring work that makes you better. Stay the course.

2. **Commitment.** Show up ready on days you feel like it and on days you do not. Your commitment should be as solid as concrete.

3. **Work ethic.** Do the extra rep. Chase improvement, not attention.

Principle 1: Leadership

Story: Running In the Rain

Let me show you how I once put my three superpowers into practice… in the pouring rain.

When my wife and I trained for half marathons, we lived by a simple rule: no excuses. Rain, cold, tired, busy, work stuff, it didn't matter. We ran.

One morning, it was coming down hard. The kind of rain that soaks you before you even make it to the end of the driveway—yeah, that kind. My wife looked at me with that "are you serious right now?" face and asked, "Are we really running outside today?"

I laughed and said, "We made a commitment, so yes."

Rocket, our schnauzer mix, perked up the moment he heard "outside." This was his jam. He loved running short stretches with us, especially in the rain. Something about it made him look completely free. Ears flapping, tongue hanging, beard dripping, paws splashing through puddles like he was auditioning for a dog-food commercial.

So there we were: two humans, one excited dog, out in the rain. Minutes in, we were soaked to the bone, shoes squishing with every step, Rocket looking like he'd just been liberated from years of captivity.

And the best part? We were laughing the whole way. No stopwatch or time goal that day. Just commitment in action.

That was leadership. Discipline. Commitment. Work ethic. Not because anyone was watching, but because we said we would.

Leaders follow through, even when they (and their dogs) are dripping wet.

LACE IT UP

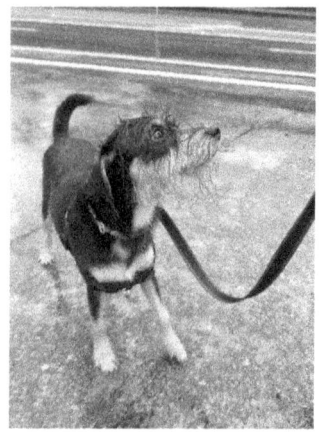

Rocket on a rainy running day.

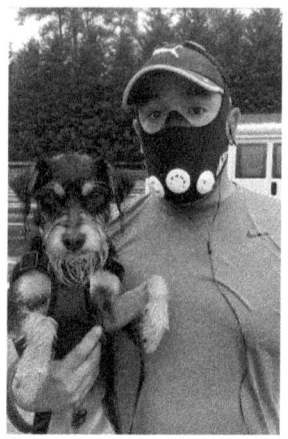

Rocket and me on a wet training day.

(with a high-altitude training mask on)

Principle 1: Leadership

Leaders Set Goals

Leaders don't just wander into the season hoping for the best. They set the target. They make it clear where the team is headed. A good goal is like GPS, it tells everyone where to go and how to get there. That's why SMART goals matter—an approach first popularized by planner George T. Doran in 1981[3]. They're specific, measurable, achievable, realistic, and timely. Basically, they're the opposite of the goals I make about eating fewer wings on wing night with the boys. (Spoiler: I never hit those.)

SMART goals give you a roadmap. Want to improve your game? Don't just say, "I'll get better at my sport." That's too vague. Instead: "In the next 90 days, I'll increase my passing accuracy to 80% in games by practicing distribution drills three times a week." Now you've got something you can track, something you can commit to, something you can actually celebrate when you hit it.

Set team goals too. The team goal is the big target. Individual goals are how each player helps hit it. Using soccer as an example, if the team goal is to make the playoffs, the keeper might focus on distribution, the winger on crossing, the striker on heading, and the coach on a new formation that fits the roster. Everyone's got their part.

And here's the kicker, leaders don't just set goals, they follow through. Write them down, track them, check in on them, and hold yourself accountable. That's how goals go from wishes to wins.

SMART goals defined:

- ✓ **Specific.** Clear target.
- ✓ **Measurable.** Numbers you can track.
- ✓ **Achievable.** Stretch, but possible.

- ✓ **Realistic.** Fits your current level.
- ✓ **Timely.** Has a deadline.

Here's a SMART Goal example I used during my training runs one year:

"In the next 90 days, I will cut 2 minutes off my 5K time by training four days a week and adding in one speed session."

Lesson: Be specific and write it down.

Pro Tip: If creating SMART goals feels overwhelming at first, start with the SCA strategy: Simple, Clear, and Actionable. This works too. And build up to SMART.

Leaders Make Decisions

You know that moment in the huddle when everyone's staring at each other like, "Sooo... what are we doing?" That's a dangerous moment. Indecision kills momentum. A team stuck waiting around is a team that's already falling behind.

That's when leaders step up. They don't always have the perfect answer, but they make a choice, they own it, and they get everyone moving in the same direction. Because here's the truth: a less-than-perfect decision made with confidence is usually better than no decision at all.

Sometimes it's picking a play when the clock is running down. Sometimes it's choosing where to eat after the game when half the squad wants tacos and the other half is chanting "pi-zza, pi-zza!" Either way, leaders decide, and when they do, people follow.

Indecision weakens a team. But decisiveness builds trust. Even if the choice doesn't work out perfectly, teammates respect the leader who had the courage to call it and the humility to adjust afterward.

Principle 1: Leadership

Good leaders:

- ✓ Gather information. Score, time, strengths, and weaknesses.
- ✓ Think through outcomes. Best case and worst case.
- ✓ Ask for advice. Coaches, teammates, sometimes even parents (imagine that)!
- ✓ Trust their instincts. Experience matters.
- ✓ Involve the team when possible. People commit to what they help build.

Huddle steps you can use:

1. State the situation. "Here is what I see..."
2. Offer two options. "Here are our choices…"
3. Ask for quick input. "What are we missing?"
4. Decide. "Here is what we are doing…"
5. Commit. "Let's lock in."

Pro Tip: Afterward, reflect on the huddle interaction. What worked? What did not? What will we change next time?

Leadership: Key Takeaways

- ✓ Leadership is more about how you act, and less about what you say.
- ✓ Energy is contagious. Make yours worth catching.
- ✓ Be the example. Effort, respect, accountability.
- ✓ Set clear goals. Keep them visible.
- ✓ Make decisions. Learn fast and move forward.

LACE IT UP

You do not need to be the coach, have a captain's band or 'C' stitched on your jersey to lead. Start with your attitude (conveniently placed as the next principle). Add effort. Treat people right. Pretty soon, the team will follow. And if they do not notice right away, keep going. Tell yourself, "Can't stop, won't stop." That is what leaders do.

Leadership: Reflections

1. Think of a teammate you look up to. What do they do that makes them a leader?

2. When was the last time you showed leadership?

3. Which leadership style (transformational, transactional, servant, democratic) feels most natural to you? Which one do you want to practice more?

4. Be honest: do you bring energy that lifts the team, or do you sometimes drain it? What can you change starting today?

Leadership: Practice

Captain Check:
- ✓ At your next practice or game, ask yourself, "If my teammates copied my effort right now, would the coach be happy?" Adjust if needed.

One Goal:
- ✓ Write down one SMART (or SCA) goal for the season. Share it with a teammate or coach (or even your parents) so they can hold you accountable.

Encourage One Teammate:
- ✓ Pick someone on your team who needs a boost. Give them one word of encouragement this week. Simple phrases like "nice work," "keep going," or "you got this" can make a big impact.

Accountability Move:
- ✓ Next time you make a mistake, own it out loud. Say *"that's on me"* or *"I'll fix it."* Then show it with your effort.

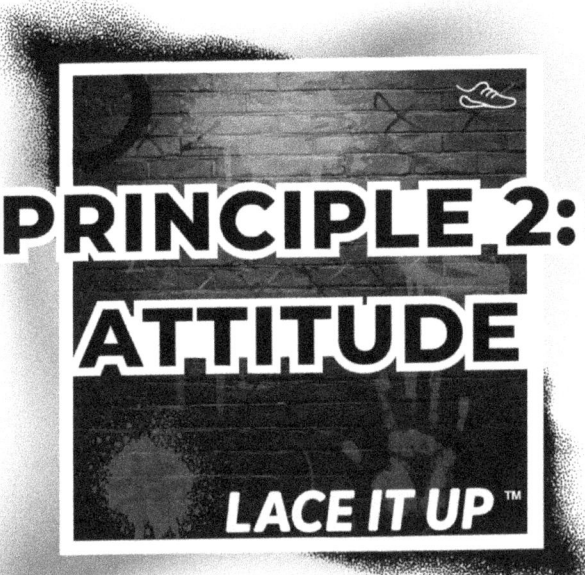

"Ability is what you're capable of doing. Motivation determines what you do. Attitude determines how well you do it."

-Lou Holtz

Principle 2: Attitude

Think about your Wi-Fi. When the signal is strong, everything flows. Games load, videos don't buffer, your texts blow up in real time. But when the signal is weak, everyone lags, you miss half the play, and people get frustrated. Your attitude works the same way. If it's strong, everyone around you connects. If it's weak, the whole team suffers. Don't be the teammate with bad service.

Your talent gets you on the field, but your attitude decides how far you go once you're there. A good attitude is like showing up every day with a clean kit, shoes tied, and ready to compete. A bad attitude? It's like showing up with your shoelaces untied and blaming the floor when you trip.

The truth is, attitude is your choice. You can't control the weather, the ref, or whether the coach runs another set of sprints. You can control how you respond. And how you respond is what your teammates, coaches, and even opponents will remember.

I tell my kids this all the time: talent might open the door, but attitude keeps you in the room. Every team has kids with skills. The ones who separate themselves are the ones who listen, bounce back, encourage others, and bring energy even on their toughest days.

Attitude also shows people who you really are when things don't go your way. It's easy to smile when you score the goal or win the game. It's much harder to smile when you miss the shot, get subbed out, or lose in overtime. That's when attitude becomes your superpower.

What Attitude Looks Like

Your attitude is your game face. It shows up before you even touch the ball. A strong attitude makes you coachable, resilient, and trustworthy. A bad one? It drags the team down like an anchor.

A good attitude looks like this:

1. You listen when coaches give feedback instead of rolling your eyes.
2. You bounce back after mistakes instead of hanging your head.
3. You encourage teammates instead of complaining.
4. You bring energy even when you are tired.

Lesson: Attitudes are contagious. Your teammates will either catch your energy or your excuses. You get to decide which one you spread.

Story: Jackson and the Power of a Positive Attitude

Picture this: Olympic Development Program tryouts. The fields are packed with the region's best, evaluators scribbling on clipboards, and parents buzzing on the sidelines. In the middle of it all is my son Jackson, 11 years old, eyes wide, nerves bouncing, ready to go all in for this opportunity. Imagine *Lose Yourself* by Eminem playing through his headphones as he prepared himself to impress the ODP staff. He was locked in.

For three days, Jackson emptied the tank. Drills, scrimmages, fitness tests, he was everywhere, hustling, encouraging,

Principle 2: Attitude

pushing himself and his teammates. By the last whistle, he was exhausted but hopeful. Then came the phone calls: his younger brother made the team for his age group right away. Jackson didn't get in.

As a dad, it gutted me. But Jackson? He dapped-up his brother, congratulated him, and celebrated like it was his own win. There were no pity parties. No excuses. Instead, he turned to me and said, "I'm not done yet. I'll keep working."

Over the next year, Jackson kept that promise. He studied his weaknesses, cheered for teammates, showed up early, and never lost his spark, even on tough days. And over time, the real shift happened: he stopped working for a spot in a program, and started chasing something bigger, unlocking a greater potential. The squad he wanted wasn't the finish line; it was a launchpad to new dreams and ambitions. The more he focused on bringing the best out of himself and others, the more doors opened. Competing clubs took notice. Scholarship offers began to roll in. But most important, he grew into someone who led by example, no matter the jersey, the team, or the outcome.

Jackson's story isn't about making or missing one team or program. It's about refusing to let disappointment write the final chapter. His attitude turned setbacks into stepping stones and, over time, his journey outgrew a single tryout.

A positive attitude won't guarantee an instant win, but it will keep you in the race for the long haul. The real victory isn't just making the roster, it's becoming the kind of person who never quits on themselves, no matter what. Let setbacks build you, not break you. The next great opportunity may just need the version of you that kept going, kept growing, and kept believing.

Why Attitude Matters

Your attitude shapes everything.

1. Coachability. A good attitude makes you easier to teach.
2. Resilience. Mistakes and losses happen. Attitude is what gets you back up.
3. Energy. Your mood impacts the team's mood.
4. Growth. Positive players keep improving. Negative ones get stuck.

Sports will test your attitude constantly. A bad call, a tough opponent, a losing streak. You can't control those things, but you can always control your response.

Mindset: The Engine of Attitude

Mindset is the way you talk to yourself when no one can hear you and three little letters can change your whole game. The three letters are Y-E-T.

"I can't do this."

Stop there, and the story is over. Add *yet*, and the story is still being written:

"I can't do this... *yet*."

"I can't dribble without looking at the ball... *yet*."

"I don't understand this play... *yet*."

"I'm not confident taking shots... *yet*."

That one word flips your attitude from fixed to growing. It's the difference between quitting and sticking with it.

Fixed vs. Growth Mindset: Two Different Games

Dr. Carol Dweck, a researcher at Stanford, spent decades studying what makes people push through setbacks. Her work on mindset is legendary and her book *Mindset: The New Psychology of Success* is a must-read in my opinion. She found that a fixed mindset says, "This is who I am. I was either born with it, or I wasn't." A growth mindset says, "I can get better if I put in the work, learn from mistakes, and stay open to feedback."[4]

Here's the truth: attitude and mindset aren't just about talent. They're about belief. If you believe you're stuck, you'll act stuck. If you believe you can grow, you'll act like growth is possible, and it usually is.

Think of it like playing two different sports:

- ✘ In the fixed-mindset game, mistakes are losses, failure feels fatal, and criticism cuts deep. You play scared.
- ✓ In the growth-mindset game, mistakes are data, failure is fuel, and feedback is a chance to level up. You play free.

Which game sounds more fun?

Why Yet Matters in Sports (and Life)

Sports are designed to test you. You'll miss scoring opportunities, drop passes, strike out, fall behind, or face someone faster, taller, or stronger. That's not bad luck, that's life. The players who thrive aren't always the most talented. They're the ones who respond with *yet*.

"I can't juggle to 100 yet."

"I haven't hit 50 consecutive free throws yet."

"I can't make top bin saves yet."

"I don't have a 25-inch vertical jump yet."

"I'm not in shape to run next year's marathon in Montana yet."

LACE IT UP

"I can't run the 40-yard dash in under 5 seconds yet."

They see the challenge as part of the process. Every "not yet" becomes a training plan, not a tombstone.

When my son Jackson started playing rec soccer, he struggled with juggling the ball. He'd get a small number of touches and the ball would hit the ground. Frustration kicked in. He said, "I can't even juggle 10 times." I reminded him: "You can't juggle 10 times *yet*. Keep working." He stayed at it.

Days later, after countless failed attempts, I heard him yell from the backyard: "I got 12!" That's *yet* in action. The skill didn't arrive in one giant leap. It grew, rep by rep, fueled by a mindset that believed growth was possible.

What a growth mindset sounds like:

"I cannot do this yet. I will adjust and keep working."

"Mistakes are data. I will use them."

"Coaching is not an attack. It is information to get better."

"Effort plus strategy beats talent that stops trying."

"Hard today means easier tomorrow."

Quick tools:

1. Yet Swap: Add "yet" to the end of the hardest sentence in your head.
2. Praise the Process: Compliment effort, focus, and tactics, not just outcomes.
3. Challenge Zone: Aim for work that is not easy and don't panic. Find the stretch.

Principle 2: Attitude

Courage: The Muscle Inside Attitude

Courage is the separator—the force that turns ordinary athletes into game-changers when it matters most. It is not the loudest voice in the room, the trash-talker, or the player banging lockers before a game. Courage is often quieter and tougher than hype. It is the grip you find on the inside, the whisper that says, "I'll try again," after failure, the choice to push forward when comfort says quit.

Some people think courage is something you either have or you do not. The truth? Courage is strength, and it is built like muscle. Every time you act instead of hide, own your mistakes, or step up when you are nervous, you make courage a little stronger. Courage burns. It makes you sore. Each "hard rep"—solving a tough problem, owning your part in a loss, risking truth in front of others—builds you up for the next test.

Weak-minded athletes blame others, make excuses, and complain when things do not go their way. Courage counters that. Courage stands up, takes responsibility, and always looks to get better. A growth mindset fuels courage. If you believe you can get stronger and improve—no matter where you start—you are willing to risk failing, willing to learn, and ready to keep moving forward during the tough moments.

Courage is the teammate who bounces back after missing a shot and says, "Let's go again." The leaders call the huddle when the team is struggling and demand more. Courage lives in athletes who refuse to hide, refuse to blame, and keep stepping up when it would be easier to disappear into the crowd.

Think of your biggest moments—pressure, doubt, adversity—they demand more than talent or hype. They demand you show up with strength, risk something, and move forward anyway. That is courage. That is the kind of inner muscle every champion trains. And the best part? You can build it every single day, even when nobody else is watching.

LACE IT UP

What courage looks like on a team:

1. Asking for the ball after a mistake. Anyone can hide after messing up. It takes courage to raise your hand and ask for another shot.

2. Owning an error out loud and fixing it. Instead of blaming, pointing fingers, or pretending it didn't happen, a courageous leader says, "That one's on me. I'll get it right next time."

3. Volunteering for a tough matchup or new position. The easy path is staying in your comfort zone. The growth path is stepping into the unknown and showing you're willing to compete anywhere.

4. Speaking up with a respectful truth when the team needs it. Courageous leaders don't stay silent when the standard is slipping. They call it out, not to embarrass but to elevate.

5. Taking or stopping the next shot, making the next tackle, doing the next sprint. Even when your legs are heavy and lungs are burning, courage is showing up for the moment that matters.

Mini-rules:

- ✓ Five-Second Countdown Rule: After a mistake, count down from 5 to 1. On 1, reset and lift off like a rocket.

- ✓ First-Rep Rule: Do the hardest drill first. Never hide from a challenge.

- ✓ One Brave Thing: Perform one courageous act at every practice or game. Small acts of courage are fine.

Why Courage Matters

Without courage, attitude crumbles the moment pressure shows up. Anyone can smile when the score is overwhelmingly in your favor. But when you're down big with minutes left? That's when courage decides if your attitude holds strong or folds.

Courage is also contagious. When one player dives for a ball, others follow. When one player steps up after a mistake, it gives the whole team permission to reset. Courage creates momentum and momentum changes games.

Lesson: Attitude is not only how you feel. It is how you think and what you do when it is hard.

Developing A Winning Attitude

Let's be honest: the goal in sports is to win. That's why we keep score, why we huddle up, and why we show up ready to battle for every inch. There's nothing wrong with you wanting to win, and there's power in developing a winning attitude from the start. A winning attitude is not about being arrogant, or thinking you're better than others. It's about showing up every day determined to give your best, compete with pride, and do the work that puts your team in position to succeed.

Winning shouldn't be a dirty word. In fact, it is why we play the game. Pro athletes and coaches are measured by wins and losses for a reason—because when the competition is real, results matter. At higher levels, if you can't help your team win, you get benched, traded, or even let go. As you grow older, sports get more competitive, and the pressure to win gets real. That's not a bad thing. It sharpens you, teaches you to handle setbacks, and rewards growth.

Rewarding everyone just for showing up and handing out participation medals might make people feel good for a moment, but it doesn't build lasting confidence or hunger. Real confidence comes from earning something—fighting for it, preparing for it, and then delivering when it counts. I believe if you want to motivate young athletes for the long run, teach them to invest in the process of getting better every day. Celebrate progress. Acknowledge the effort. But also be clear: results matter too. Not everyone wins the trophy, and that's okay. Use it. Let it fuel your fire to improve.

A winning attitude means you want to be part of a team that chases excellence together. It means you bounce back from loss, learn from mistakes, and come back stronger. Coaches notice the players who treat every practice, every drill, and every game as a chance to win—not just the scoreboard, but the small battles: every challenge, every hustle play, every decision to give a little more.

Do not let anyone tell you that wanting to win is wrong, or that it is enough to just show up and go through the motions. A winning attitude is about striving, growing, and believing that your work can tip the scales. If you want to go far—in sports or in life—make this your standard: strive to win the right way, invest in your journey, and never apologize for your drive to be the best you can be. That is the mindset champions build, and it starts with how you play today.

The Bad Attitude Trap

Every team has them. The players with bad attitudes. They're not always bad kids, but their behavior can drag everyone else down. Attitude is contagious, and negative attitudes spread the fastest.

Principle 2: Attitude

Most common "bad attitudes" in sports:

1. **The Complainer**
   Finds fault with everything: the refs, the field, the coach, the weather. "It's too hot." "These drills are boring." "This ref hates us." Complaining doesn't fix problems. It just drains energy.

2. **The Blamer**
   Never owns mistakes. Every bad pass, every goal, every loss is someone else's fault. Blamers don't learn. If it's never their responsibility, they never improve.

3. **The Sulker**
   Subbed out? Head down. Missed a shot? Hands up. Their body language screams, "I give up." And when they slump, the team slumps too.

4. **The Quitter**
   Shuts down when things get tough. Down a few goals? They stop hustling. Behind on fitness runs? They coast. Quitting isn't about losing the game. It's about losing the fight inside you.

5. **The Drama Starter**
   Stirs up gossip, arguments, or conflict. Eye rolls, side comments, or makes back-and-forth chatter that poisons the huddle or locker room. Drama destroys trust, and trust is the glue of every good team.

These attitudes are easy to catch. Often, a bad attitude hides fear. Replace fear with a plan: mindset tools + one brave action.

Pro Tip: Don't be the teammate who makes practice feel heavier the second they walk in.

LACE IT UP

How to Handle Bad Attitudes

At some point, you'll be teammates with one (or more) of these players. You can't always control who's on your team.

How to respond to bad attitudes:

1. Model the opposite. Be the encourager, the listener, the hard worker.

2. Don't take the bait. When someone complains or blames, don't pile on. Redirect your energy to the game or practice.

3. Encourage quietly. A simple "You got this" can pull a teammate out of a slump.

4. Stay focused. Their attitude is theirs. Yours is yours.

Lesson: Bad attitudes will always be around. The choice is whether you catch them... or stop them from spreading.

Analogy: The Mirror Effect

Your attitude is like a mirror, and your team is always watching.

Walk onto the field with your shoulders slumped, head down, and a storm cloud over your head? Watch the energy drain out of everyone around you—they'll mirror that slump right back. But show grit after a mistake, clap your hands, lift your chin, and fire off a "We got this, next play!"—suddenly, watch the whole squad snap back to life.

It's not just the words, it's the vibe. Blame others and negativity spreads like wildfire, one bad mood can take down the whole bench. Show hustle, keep hustling, and your teammates will lean in and match your energy. Confidence, resilience, accountability, those things bounce around a team like a ball in a drill.

Principle 2: Attitude

Here's the truth: you set the tone. When you show courage, your team finds theirs. When you lift others, you all rise. You get back what you put out. Make your mirror worth reflecting.

Story: The Toxic Parent

Every coach has "that parent" at some point. One season, mine couldn't keep quiet on the sideline. He hadn't played beyond rec soccer, but was convinced he knew more about the game than a coach with a professional background and a closet full of old jerseys. His running commentary at games was as predictable as the traffic I dealt with leaving the fields after practice.

Every whistle, every water break, there it was—the sound of fresh complaints drifting down the sideline. The classics?

"The coach doesn't know what he's doing."

"This formation is all wrong. Honestly, nobody uses it anymore—this is joke!"

"Why is that player even here – he's terrible!"

"If my kid doesn't start, we're quitting the club. I know people 'ABC academy,' you know."

At first, none of this seemed to faze the player. The kid was everything you wanted—optimistic, respectful, a great teammate. But week after week, that steady drip of negativity started to wear him down. Soon, the player began to echo his dad's frustration: rolling eyes at the coach, snapping at teammates, and doubting himself any time things went wrong. I felt bad for because the kid was a victim of his dad's negative influence.

By the end of the season, both father and son left the club in dramatic fashion—think less "mic drop" and more

LACE IT UP

"sideline stomp." Here's the wild part: after they left, the team's chemistry took off like someone finally aired out the locker room. The smiles came back. Practice felt lighter. And guess what? Our team actually got better.

Here's the truth: attitude is contagious. When a parent's negativity spills over, kids pick it up quick. And the best winning teams? They build each other up, not tear each other down. If you are a parent and find yourself slipping into this mode, check yourself—you might just be the plot twist your kid's team doesn't need. And if you're the player with a parent like this, pull them aside and have a private conversation. Give them the feedback in a respectful way and ask to see changes in their behavior. If they support the LACE IT UP principles, they'll adjust and be better because they care and want to support you.

Lesson: Parents' attitudes matter, but you still get to choose your own.

Story: The Two Dogs Inside Us

There's an old tale about a boy who was angry and complaining after a tough loss. His grandfather told him, "Inside every person, there are two dogs. One dog is negative — jealous, lazy, angry, always making excuses. The other dog is positive — grateful, hardworking, focused, and full of energy. These dogs are always fighting. And do you know which one wins?"

The boy thought for a moment and asked, "Which one?"
The grandfather replied, "The one you feed."

Now, that's the classic version. But if you're like me, you're probably picturing two dogs sitting at your dinner table fighting over a plate of chicken nuggets. One's grumpy, saying, "Why do we even have practice tonight?" The other's smiling, saying, "Nice, extra reps."

Principle 2: Attitude

Here's the truth: you're feeding one of those dogs every single day. Skip reps at practice? The negative dog just got a Happy Meal. Encourage a teammate after a mistake? The positive dog gets a milkshake. Roll your eyes at your coach? The negative dog just gained an advantage. Reset and say, "It's okay, next play." The positive dog just got stronger.

The dog you feed becomes the one that runs the show. Keep feeding the negative dog, and it grows into a Bulldog that takes over your attitude. Keep feeding the positive dog, and it grows into a Great Dane that chases the negative one down until it's nothing more than a yappy little Chihuahua.

Lesson: Feed the positive dog, or the negative one will eat your lunch.

LACE IT UP

Attitude: Key Takeaways

- ✓ Attitude is your game face. Wear it before the whistle.
- ✓ Growth mindset fuels attitude: add 'yet', treat mistakes as data.
- ✓ Courage is part of attitude: do one brave thing every day.
- ✓ Your attitude spreads fast. Make people catch your energy, not your excuses.
- ✓ You cannot control everything. You can always control your response.

Attitude: Reflections

1. Where did you use a growth mindset this week? Where did a fixed mindset show up?
2. What is one brave action you avoided recently? What will it look like to do it next time?
3. When was the last time you reset fast after a mistake? What helped?
4. Think of a teammate with a great attitude. What can you copy?
5. Which dog are you feeding more often, and how will you change the menu?

Attitude: Practice

Yet Swap:
- ✓ Write one skill you cannot do yet. Add a plan with two steps for this week.

Courage Reps:
- ✓ Do one brave thing in each practice or game. Ask for the ball, take the tough mark, speak up.

Reset Button:
- ✓ After a mistake, clap once and say "Next play." Countdown five seconds, then take off to the next thing.

Positive Shoutout:
- ✓ Encourage at least one teammate every practice or game this week.

Gratitude Drill:
- ✓ After practice, jot one thing you are grateful for. Gratitude fuels attitude.

LACE IT UP

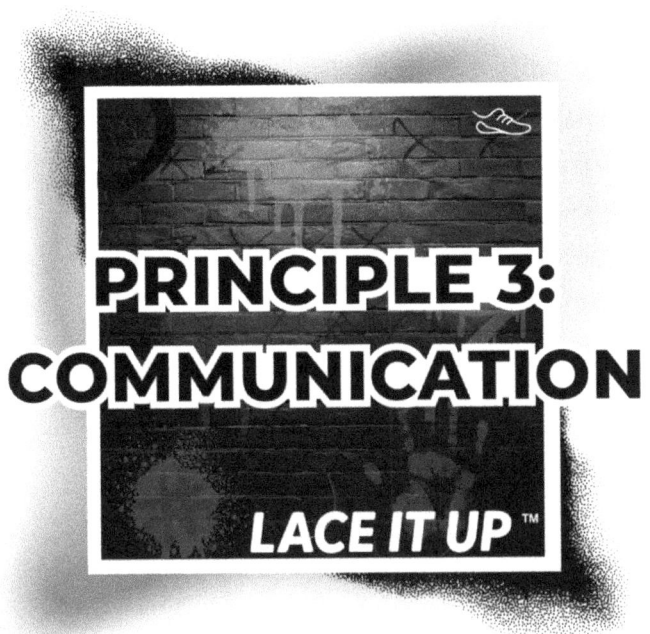

"Effective teamwork begins and ends with communication."

– Mike Krzyzewski
(coach K)

Principle 3:

Communication

Think about the best teams you've ever seen. They look connected, almost like they're moving with one mind. No confusion, no hesitation, just smooth flow. That doesn't happen by accident. It happens because they talk. Constantly.

But here's the thing: most young athletes confuse talking with communicating. Talking is just sound. Communication has purpose. It's the signal in the noise. It's the difference between a bunch of players running around yelling random stuff and a team that's locked in, sharp, and organized.

I tell my boys all the time: silence is the enemy of teamwork. Communication is like a pair of wireless headphones. When the connection is clear, the music flows. Every beat, every lyric, smooth and in sync. You nod your head and everything feels right.

But what if the Bluetooth signal keeps cutting out? The sound lags and you hear static. It's frustrating. You can't lock in. That's what happens on a team when people stop talking. The rhythm is gone. The flow is broken.

Great communication keeps the connection strong, so the whole team is on the same beat.

LACE IT UP

If you don't speak up, bad things happen. Teammates collide. Players mark the wrong opponent. Missed chances pile up. Confidence slips. A team without communication is like a band playing with no conductor — each person might be talented, but together it sounds like chaotic noise.

Here's the other side of it: communication builds trust. When your teammate calls, "I've got your back!" you believe them. When you hear, "Man on!" you react faster. When your captain shouts, "Next play, we got this," you feel your energy rise. Words create confidence. Words carry leadership. Words change the whole atmosphere of a game.

And communication isn't just for the moments when you're directly involved with the ball. The best communicators talk when they're far away from the play in motion. They keep teammates locked in, aware, and motivated. They don't disappear when things get tough — their voice is the rope that pulls the team forward.

The truth? Every team has a choice: chaos or connection. Noise or communication. Teammates who keep their voices to themselves, or teammates who share what they see, what they feel, and what the team needs.

The great teams pick connection. They build a culture where talking isn't optional, it's expected. They know communication is not just a tool — it's oxygen.

Strong communication looks like:

1. Calling for the ball so teammates know where you are.
2. Giving encouragement after mistakes: "Next play, we got this."
3. Directing teammates with quick cues: "Man on!" or "Switch!"

Principle 3: Communication

4. Staying vocal even when the ball is far away, so the team stays organized.

Here's the truth: when communication disappears, chaos shows up. Teammates crash into each other. Defenders mark the wrong player. Chances get missed. Silence is the enemy of teamwork.

Story: Carson Finds His Voice

When my son Carson was 8, we made the leap from rec soccer to club soccer. My wife and I didn't grow up playing soccer, so we were learning the game right alongside our boys.

At our very first pre-season tournament, the coach asked the team who wanted to play goalkeeper. He told the boys, "I need someone brave, because keeper is the hardest position. It's not for everyone." I sat quietly on the sideline praying my son wouldn't raise his hand. I knew enough to know goalkeepers live a tough life. Everyone remembers the goals you don't stop, not the saves you make.

But of course, Carson's hand shot straight up. And just like that, we had ourselves a keeper.

Poor Carson had no idea what he was doing. We lost every game that weekend. The coach encouraged him though, praising his courage and telling us to get him into goalkeeper training. He promised Carson would improve. And the first thing we did after that tournament was pull up YouTube tutorials and study pro keepers. Not just how they dove or caught the ball, but how they communicated.

That's where the magic happened. Carson learned quickly that a keeper can't stay quiet. He had to be the eyes and voice of the defense. Even when the ball was far away, he had to keep his teammates locked in: "Push up!" "Mark your man!" "High press!" "Drop!" "Well done boys!" "Jog it off!"

At just 8 years old, it was rare to hear a keeper so vocal. But Carson embraced it. Communication became his superpower and differentiator. His skills improved with reps and training, sure, but his voice, his ability to direct and encourage, made him stand out. Coaches noticed. Teammates trusted him. And communication became the thing that turned a nervous kid who raised his hand into a natural leader on the field.

Lesson: Communication is more than words — it's leadership in action.

Story: Megan Rapinoe's Voice

That's one kid's story. Now let's zoom out to the biggest stage in the world.

Picture the scene: 2019 Women's World Cup. Millions watching. One mistake could end the U.S. team's run. The pressure was insane. Players looked tight. Nerves were high.

Enter Megan Rapinoe. She wasn't just running the wing — she was running her mouth, in the best way possible. Constantly. I imagine if she were mic'd, you could hear her saying:

"Push up!" "We got this!" "Keep the ball moving!"

She wasn't communicating just to be loud. She was steadying her teammates. You could see it on their faces. The younger players looked to her, fed off her energy, and settled into the game.

And then came the goals. Rapinoe scored clutch penalties, celebrated with arms wide open, and became the heartbeat of the team. But if you ask her teammates, it wasn't just the goals that carried them. It was her presence, her constant voice reminding them they belonged on the biggest stage.

Principle 3: Communication

By the end of the tournament, the U.S. lifted the trophy again. Rapinoe won the Golden Ball and Golden Boot. But in her interviews, she didn't brag — she praised the team.

Lesson: Great players don't just play — they communicate.

Why Communication Matters

Whether it's a kid in goal or a star on the world stage, communication is the glue that holds teams together. Without it, even talented players fall apart.

Here's why communication matters:

1. Trust. Teammates believe in each other when voices stay steady.
2. Awareness. Talking keeps everyone locked in on their roles.
3. Encouragement. Positive words fuel effort when things get tough.
4. Problem-Solving. Communication clears confusion before it becomes chaos.

Lesson: Silence doesn't win games. Teams that talk, win.

Analogy: The Online Game Squad

Communication is just like teaming up in Fortnite, Rocket League, or Call of Duty. Everyone joins in, ready for battle, headset on, and the mission is clear: work together, watch each other's backs, and chase the win. You call out enemies. You shout when you need help. You drop "it's over here" or "cover me, I'm reviving." Play as a team and your chances skyrocket.

But imagine your mic goes down. Suddenly, the plan falls apart. Your squad splits up, someone gets ambushed, two teammates rush the same side, and the one person with a working headset is left yelling into the void "what is going on, can anybody hear me?" Then game over. You had no chance against a team that was dialed in and talking. Silence on the squad is chaos. Everyone's guessing. Nobody knows when the trap is coming or where to regroup.

In team sports, it works exactly the same way. Talent helps, but talent in silence is wasted. When athletes share calls, encourage each other, and react fast, confusion disappears and the game flows. The best teams "play with mics on," talking, listening, solving problems together in real time.

Lesson: Mute your voice and you play solo, even when you're surrounded by teammates. If you want to win in team sports or on your favorite game, keep your headset charged, your channel open, and your squad connected. That's how teams move as one.

Active Listening: The Secret Weapon

Talking is only half the equation. Too many athletes get stuck in broadcast mode, shouting instructions, cheering, or giving advice without actually picking up what's coming back. But what about the teams that really click? They have players who listen with purpose. Active listening is what turns noise into understanding.

Here's what it looks like. An active listener locks eyes when a teammate or coach talks. They nod, echo back, and check for clarity with a quick "so what you're saying is... right?" or "got it, drop back and press." They don't just wait for their turn to talk; they tune in and make sure the message truly lands.

Active listening is like fielding a pass. If you're lazy with your footwork, you lose possession. If you're lazy with your ears, the play breaks down and the whole team pays. Every leader, from captains to quiet fill-in players, knows: the best way

Principle 3: Communication

to earn trust is to prove you're really hearing the people around you.

What separates a good listener? It's doing all of this, even under pressure. When the coach gives last-minute instructions, when a teammate's feedback stings, or when the stadium noise is thunderous, good teammates block out the static and catch what matters.

Do this, and you build credibility. Teammates come to you after a mistake because they know you listen. Coaches give you bigger responsibilities. You become the center of the team's communication chain, the one who holds everything together.

Not everyone is born with great listening skills, but everyone can get better with practice. Next time someone talks, pause. Repeat back what you heard. Ask a clarifying question. Watch how quickly your relationships and your team's on-field performance start to level up. Active listening is consistently ranked among the most important communication skills by successful athletes and coaches[5].

Active listening looks like this:
1. Eyes up when a teammate or coach speaks.
2. Nodding or giving a quick "Got it."
3. Asking questions if you're not clear.
4. Adjusting your play to match what was said.

Lesson: Don't just be loud. Be the teammate who listens, adjusts, and always delivers the message.

Story: The Over-Eager Sideline Parent

Of course, sometimes communication goes too far. Every team has that parent on the sideline. The one who yells every five seconds. The one who thinks they're helping… but usually aren't.

For a while, that parent was me.

When Carson first started playing goalkeeper, I was so passionate, so invested, that I thought it was my job to coach him from the sideline. Every game you'd hear my voice carrying across the field:

"Great save, Carson!"

"There's only one mode. BEASTMODE!"

"Stay on your line!"

"Tell them what you see, tell them what you need!"

"You have to be better than that."

"You have to close the gap in 1 v 1 moments."

I thought I was helping. I thought my words were keeping him sharp. But the truth? I was distracting him. Instead of focusing on his positioning, his communication with defenders, or listening to his coach, he had to deal with me yelling a nonstop stream of affirmations, instructions, and criticism.

Finally, one game, the coach had enough. He turned to the sideline, raised his voice, and said: "Do not coach the players please. Thank you!"

In an instant, I felt every parent's eyes on me. My face burned red. I sat back in my chair, embarrassed but also humbled. I realized something: I had crossed the line. Cheering is one thing. Coaching from the sideline is another. My job wasn't to coach; it was to parent. My role was encouragement, not direction.

It stung in the moment, but that coach did me a favor. He communicated clearly. He set expectations. And because of that, I learned how to be a better sideline parent.

Principle 3: Communication

Lesson: Sometimes the best communication is knowing when not to speak.

Giving and Receiving Feedback

Feedback is one of the toughest, most powerful tools in sports. It can sting, bruise the ego, and leave you frustrated for a moment. But skip feedback and you skip growth. On every great team, feedback is how players get sharper, teams get tighter, and mistakes become springboards.

The difference between good teams and great ones isn't just what they say; it's how they listen, absorb, and act on the hard truths. Learning how to give feedback, clear, honest, and supportive, matters just as much as learning how to take it. Players and coaches who master both won't just improve; they'll earn trust, respect, and lasting confidence.

Good feedback turns losses into lessons, frustration into fuel, and setbacks into comebacks. It's not always easy, but it's always necessary. The key is learning how to give it and receive it without ego. That's how you build coaches, captains, and teammates every team wants more of.

Good feedback is:
- ✓ Specific: "Mark #10 tighter,"
- ✓ Supportive: "You got this, next time,"
- ✓ Timely: Given right after the moment.

Bad feedback is:
- ✗ Not Specific: "Play better defense."
- ✗ Not Supportive: "You're terrible."
- ✗ Not Timely: Given days later.

LACE IT UP

Receiving feedback looks like:
- ✓ Don't argue. Just listen.
- ✓ Say "Got it." and show appreciation and gratitude.
- ✓ Show you heard by adjusting your play.

Lesson: Feedback is fuel. Take it in and burn brighter.

Resolving Conflicts

Conflict is the price of caring. When you put your heart into a team, frustration and disagreement are bound to show up. Passions run high, tempers flare, and sometimes even the closest teammates butt heads. Do you want the truth? If everyone agrees all the time, somebody isn't telling the truth, or the team isn't pushing hard enough. Sit with that thought for a moment.

The best teams refuse to let conflict linger like a shadow in the locker room. They don't pretend problems away or sweep them under the rug. They face them head on, handle them like teammates, not rivals, and come out stronger on the other side. Growth lives on the other side of a tough conversation. I know that might sound strange, but I'm asking you to trust me here.

Every good team environment breed honesty, not just harmony. Real trust is built when players can disagree, resolve it, and move forward together. Handled right, conflict isn't a setback; it's a springboard to deeper trust, better chemistry, and greater success.

Steps to resolve conflicts:
1. Cool down. Don't try to fix things while angry. Give the oatmeal time to cool before you place a spoonful in your mouth.

Principle 3: Communication

2. Talk it out. Pull the teammate aside and be honest. Create a private space for a healthy dialogue.
3. Listen back. Hear their side too.
4. Move forward. Leave the issue on the field once it's addressed.

Conflicts are like tangled shoelaces. Ignore them, and they trip you up. Work them out, and you can keep running.

Lesson: Teams that handle conflict build stronger trust.

Encouraging Unity and Inclusion

A team isn't just a group of athletes wearing the same jersey. The best teams feel like family, everyone belongs, everyone matters, and every voice gets heard. The secret isn't talent or highlight reels; it's how players use their words to pull everyone into the circle.

Great teammates look for moments to build bridges. New kid on the roster? They're welcomed, not ignored. Quiet players who hesitate, speedy scorers who grab all the attention, unity means nobody feels left out. Inclusion is built one small gesture at a time: a nickname, a high-five, a simple "nice work" after a tough drill.

Communication is the spark. Every "good job," every inside joke, every word of encouragement tightens the bond. When players connect off the field, trust flourishes on it. Chemistry grows, mistakes shrink, and winning starts to feel like something everyone helped create. Strong teams aren't just skilled, they're united. And unity happens one conversation, one celebration, one shared moment at a time.

Ways to insert good communication:
1. Learn everyone's name, even the new players.

LACE IT UP

2. Celebrate small wins: "Nice pass!" "Nice shot" or "Great hustle!"
3. Share the ball. Literally and verbally. Don't freeze out teammates.
4. Watch your tone. Common mistake: yelling at someone isn't the same as motivating them.
5. Always provide a warm welcome for new players on the team.

Lesson: Communication builds chemistry. When everyone feels included, the team gets stronger.

Story: The Silent Game

One practice, a team thought they were in for a simple challenge. Coach called everyone in. "For the next five minutes," she said, "play in total silence. No talking. No calling. No signals. Just play." A few kids grinned, some rolled their eyes, most laughed, thinking it sounded easy.

Then the whistle blew. Suddenly, it was like the whole squad forgot how to play together. Passes landed in empty space. Teammates collided. Shots came out of nowhere but no one was ready to rebound or cover. Communication evaporated, chemistry was gone, and suddenly the field of play felt twice as big and ten times as confusing.

You could see frustration mounting, arms in the air, panicked glances, gestures that meant nothing without words. It was chaos. For five long minutes, the drill kept running: wrong moves, missed chances, teammates bumping into each other like they'd never practiced a day in their lives.

Finally, coach blew the whistle. Everyone froze, exhausted and baffled. "See?" she said, voice cutting through the

Principle 3: Communication

silence. "That's what happens when you don't talk. No communication, no connection, no team."

In that moment, you could see understanding click. Players looked around and realized it wasn't talent or hard work that broke down, it was simply not speaking up. From that day, the team got louder and smarter. Nobody wanted another silent five minutes.

Lesson: Communication isn't optional for a team. It's oxygen. Without it, no matter how skilled you are, you can't breathe life into teamwork.

Communication: Key Takeaways

- ✓ Communication is more than talking — it's listening, too.
- ✓ Great communicators give clear, positive, and timely messages.
- ✓ Silence leads to chaos. Talking keeps teams organized and confident.
- ✓ Words can lift a team or tear it down. Choose wisely.

Communication: Reflections

1. Think about a time your team struggled because nobody talked. What happened?
2. Who's the best communicator on your team? What makes them effective?
3. Do you listen as well as you talk? Be honest.
4. How can you use communication to build trust on your team this week?

Communication: Practice

Three Shoutouts Drill:
- ✓ In your next game, commit to three purposeful shoutouts per half. One for direction, one for encouragement, one for awareness.

Communication Hack:
- ✓ When a coach or captain gives instructions, repeat it back so teammates know you heard and to encourage more communication amongst the team.

Encourage One:
- ✓ Pick a teammate who struggles with confidence. Give them two positive shoutouts in practice this week.

Conflict Reset:
- ✓ If you argue with a teammate, pull them aside after practice and clear it up.

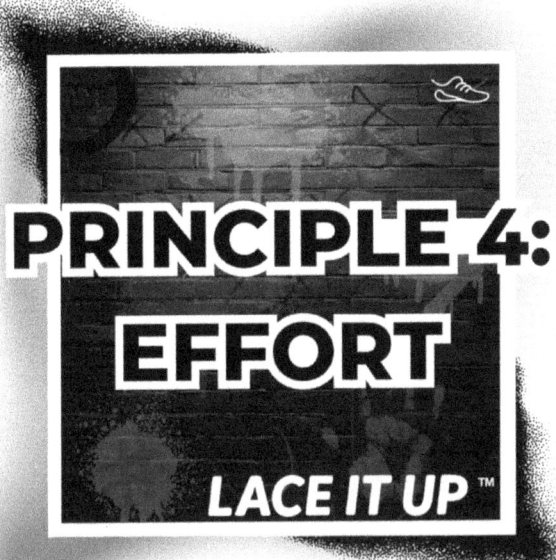

"There may be people that have more talent than you, but there's no excuse for anyone to work harder than you do."

– Derek Jeter

Principle 4: Effort

Every athlete's journey starts and ends with effort. It isn't the flash of brilliance or the high-adrenaline moments, no, that's intensity, and its time will come. Effort is different. It's the unglamorous grind, the quiet work ethic that gets overlooked and undervalued. Effort is what you do when the lights are off, when the coach isn't looking, when there's nothing but your own standard to meet.

Effort is the choice to show up every day and give what you have, even when you're not feeling it. There's no scoreboard for effort, but there's a reputation, a standard, an expectation. Teammates notice who hustles in warmups, who never coasts through drills, and who keeps moving when most have stopped. Is that you? If not, it should be. The impact isn't in any one moment, it's in showing up, over and over, until your effort becomes a habit.

Real effort isn't about being the loudest or the most talented. It's about being reliable and tough. It's about being the one anyone can count on for maximum hustle no matter the situation. Sometimes it's sprinting after a ball you might not reach, sometimes it's staying late for one extra rep, sometimes simply refusing to quit. On the hardest days, your effort may just mean getting through the next drill with focus and pride.

Effort means you refuse to settle for "good enough." You take accountability for your role, whether starter or support. When you bring effort, you raise not just your level but everyone else's. It's the baseline and the floor all teams stand on.

Intensity is fuel for the big moments, but effort is the engine that never stops. It's the commitment that carries you from practice to game to championship, building the foundation for every win and every comeback. You don't get to choose your talent, but you always choose your effort.

So before chasing bursts of intensity, master the constant pursuit. Make effort your trademark. Let it be what teammates and coaches remember, because it's what will set you apart every single day.

What Effort Looks Like

Effort is the fuel that drives everything else: leadership, attitude, communication, skill. You can't control your height, your speed, or your natural talent. But you can always control your effort.

Effort looks like this:

1. Sprinting after a ball you probably won't get, but trying anyway.
2. Showing up early and staying late.
3. 'Emptying the tank' and giving your all in the last minute of the game, not just the first.
4. Playing through discomfort (smartly, not dangerously) because your team needs you.

Lesson: Effort doesn't always guarantee you'll win, but a lack of effort almost always guarantees you'll lose.

Principle 4: Effort

Story: Jackson's Rising Stars Tournament

It was late May, and the sun was beating down. A one-day Rising Stars soccer tournament, three to five games packed into a single day. Our team came in as underdogs. The team was made up of kids from his academy team, led by a coach who didn't play the sport professionally or even recreationally for that matter. I was the coach; the team was called Born BEASTMODE and nobody expected much.

But Jackson did.

From the first whistle, he was determined. He ran, pressed, fought for every ball. He scored goals and celebrated with his teammates. When I tried to sub him out, he shook his head. "No Dad, uh coach, don't sub me out, my team needs me."

By the semifinal, you could see the exhaustion on every player's face. The game went into penalty kicks. Jackson buried his shot, the team advanced, and everyone collapsed in relief.

Here's the kicker: the final started immediately after that grueling semi. No rest. No break. We were drained. The other team was fresh. We fought, but we lost. Though we had finalists' medals around our necks, we felt like champions. We walked off the pitch with our heads high and felt extremely proud of our accomplishments.

That night when we got home, Jackson looked pale. We took his temperature and learned he had a fever. The next day, the doctor told us he had a double ear and sinus infection.

He never said a word about feeling sick. The morning of the tournament he mentioned being a little tired and having a runny nose. My son gave everything he had that day. His effort and refusal to quit were infectious. His teammates felt it. I felt it.

LACE IT UP

Lesson: Effort doesn't always lead to a trophy, but it always leaves a mark.

Story: Michael Jordan's "Flu Game"

Now let's zoom out to one of the greatest effort stories in sports history.

It was June 11, 1997. The Chicago Bulls were tied 2–2 in the NBA Finals against the Utah Jazz. Game 5 was massive. Win, and you're one step closer to a championship. Lose, and you're on the ropes.

Michael Jordan could barely stand.

He was pale, drenched in sweat, weak with fever and dehydration. Trainers said he looked exhausted just walking. Most players would've sat out. Nobody would've blamed him.

But Jordan suited up anyway.

From the opening minutes, you could see the pain. He leaned on teammates during timeouts. He gasped for air after every possession. The Jazz tried to wear him down.

But effort isn't about how you feel. It's about what you choose to give.

And Jordan chose to give everything.

He played 44 minutes, scored 38 points, and carried his team when they needed him most. With the game tied late, he buried a three-pointer that crushed the Jazz's spirit. When the final buzzer sounded, Jordan collapsed into teammate Scottie Pippen's arms — an image burned into sports history.

The Bulls went on to win the series and the championship. But ask anyone who watched, and they'll tell you the title was sealed in Game 5.

Principle 4: Effort

Lesson: Champions don't just shine when it's easy. They shine when it costs them everything.

Bridging the Stories

Now, Jackson's Rising Stars tournament didn't have millions of fans or TV cameras. But effort is effort. Whether it's in a packed arena or a small local field, giving everything you have inspires the people around you. That's the power of effort.

Why Effort Matters

Effort is the ultimate game-changer. Coaches crave it, teammates respect it, and opponents fear it because it's the one thing nobody can take away or out-talent. You can't control your height, your genes, or what team you start on, but effort is always yours to give.

Top-tier programs are built on sweat, hustle, and the little wins that stack up every practice. The best part? Effort pays out every single time, whether you're the star or the last player off the bench. Anyone can choose to leave the field tired and proud, and that's what sets real competitors apart from the rest.

Effort builds:

1. Consistency. Effort every day leads to steady improvement.

2. Resilience. Effort helps you push through fatigue, failure, and setbacks.

3. Respect. Coaches and teammates notice hustle, even when the scoreboard doesn't.

4. Momentum. When one player gives max effort, it spreads through the team.

LACE IT UP

Lesson: Talent sets the ceiling, but effort builds the floor.

The Effort Spectrum

Effort isn't just an on/off switch, it's a whole range, from invisible to unstoppable. Every team, every practice, every game, you'll find players all over the map. Some just show up, some coast until they're watched, some bring real hustle, and a few rare ones go all out, all the time.

The truth is, effort isn't a mystery. You can spot it in a heartbeat. You know who only works when the coach stares, and you know the one who picks up teammates, chases every play, and never takes a rep off. In sports and in life, where you land on the effort spectrum is always your choice.

Minimal Effort

✘ This player jogs through drills, avoids contact, and does the bare minimum to not get yelled at. They "show up," but that's about it.
   Minimum effort fools nobody. Coaches and teammates see it.

Situational Effort

✘ This player turns it on when the coach is watching or when the ball is at their feet. But as soon as attention shifts, they relax. They only hustle when it benefits them.
   Situational effort makes you look good sometimes, but never makes the team better.

Consistent Effort

✓ This player gives steady energy every practice, every drill, every game. You can rely on them. They don't take plays off.

Principle 4: Effort

Extra Effort

- ✓ This is the player who goes above and beyond. They chase the lost ball, cheer for teammates, stay after practice for one more rep. They don't just raise their own game; they raise everyone else's too.

Lesson: Consistency is effort's best friend. Steady effort builds steady improvement. Extra effort is contagious; it spreads and lifts the whole team.

Story: The Team Manager Who Refused to Do the Minimum

In the early years of my boy's academy soccer journey, parents volunteered as team managers. On paper, the job was simple: enter schedules in the team app, communicate game details, coordinate hotels for tournaments, and handle uniform orders. Basically, take the admin work off the coach's plate so they could focus on coaching.

My first impressions of team managers? Honestly, not great. Too many seemed more interested in having the "title" or cozying up to the coach than actually serving the team. Communication was sloppy, questions went unanswered, and parents were often confused about travel logistics or game schedules.

One season, my son's coach pulled me aside: "Would you be willing to step in as Team Manager? Our current manager is leaving, and we need someone to finish the season." He gave the impression that all I needed to do was the bare minimum to help get us to the end of the season.

I agreed, but here's the thing: I don't do minimums.

The coach gave me the basics: just keep parents informed and help with logistics. But once I understood the role was really about freeing the coach and supporting the team, I got to work.

I started proactively sending weather updates the night before games and gave recommendations on how to layer up when needed.

I wrote a "Parent Tips and Best Practices" guide to cut down sideline drama.

I organized team gatherings to boost morale.

At the end of every season, I had every player record a thank-you video for the coach, combined them into a highlight reel, and surprised the coach with a QR code linked to the video inside a card with a team donation.

Before long, other coaches were calling me to manage their teams. At one point, I was managing four teams at once, two of which my sons played on. Eventually my boys aged out of teams needing team managers, but even then, I found ways to keep helping the club.

Why? Because effort isn't just about running harder on the field. It's about taking ownership wherever you can. Doing more than what's asked. Looking for ways to make things better.

Lesson: Minimum effort meets low expectations. Maximum effort changes the game.

Analogy: The Gas Tank

Think of effort like a gas tank. Some days, you wake up with your tank totally full, you feel strong, rested, and every effort feels easy. On other days, you show up drained. Maybe you had a tough week, maybe the school day wore you down, maybe you didn't sleep well, maybe life just hits hard and you roll in running on fumes.

Principle 4: Effort

But here's the deal: you always get to choose how much you give from whatever's left in the tank. You control the pedal. Nobody else can decide for you whether to coast or to press down and give everything you've got, even if "everything" feels like less than yesterday.

You don't have to be at 100% to act like it. Let's say you show up at practice only feeling 60%. If you give all 60%, that's full effort for that day. Coaches and teammates will notice, because the hardest workers are often the ones who keep going when it would be easier to hold back.

Effort isn't about waiting until you're at your best. It's about showing up, using whatever fuel you've got, and emptying the tank for your team, your goals, and your own growth. Every drop counts. The best players gauge success not by how much they start with, but by how much they give away.

You might not be at 100%, but if you give 100% of what you have, that's effort.

Lesson: Effort isn't about how much you start with; it's about how much you give. Coaches love the player who empties the tank, especially on the days it isn't easy.

Story: The Empty Bleachers

Confession: I wasn't supposed to be at basketball practice. I was just a teenager hunting for the fastest way out of school, about to take my secret shortcut through the gym. Instantly, I stumbled onto the slowest-moving group of basketball players you've ever seen. It looked like a zombie apocalypse, nobody talking, no energy, everyone shuffling around like their shoes were made of concrete. It was like the slow-motion scenes from The Matrix, even though those movies hadn't been made yet.

The coach must have channeled his inner movie director, blowing a whistle loud enough to wake the janitor. He growled, "Wake up! Let's do it again. Only this time, pretend the bleachers are packed, stacked with college scouts, pro coaches, and all your girlfriends. Let's see if your effort changes?"

Suddenly, it was like someone swapped water bottles for rocket fuel. Players sprinted, voices echoed, bodies flying everywhere. I was half tempted to yell out my own encouragement, "Great hustle! That's what's up!" before remembering I was just a guy trying to get home, and not a scout.

Lesson: If your energy only shows up for an audience, you're playing the wrong game. Effort should never depend on who's watching, even if it's just a kid cutting through the gym looking for a shortcut.

Effort: Key Takeaways

- ✓ Effort is the one thing you can control, every time.
- ✓ Max effort doesn't always win games, but it always earns respect.
- ✓ Effort is contagious — when you give it, others catch it.
- ✓ Don't pace yourself with excuses. Empty the tank.

Effort: Reflections

1. Think about your last practice. Did you give maximum effort, or did you coast?
2. Who on your team gives consistent effort? How does it affect everyone else?
3. Have you ever surprised yourself by pushing harder than you thought you could?
4. What excuses stop you from giving full effort?

Effort: Practice

Last Sprint Best Sprint:
- ✓ At your next practice, make your final sprint your fastest. Prove you can finish strong.

Extra Rep Challenge:
- ✓ Stay after practice for one extra rep of your weakest skill.

Teammate Fuel:
- ✓ Find a tired teammate and encourage them to push.

Effort Journal:
- ✓ Write down one time each day you gave extra effort, even off the field (school, chores, family).

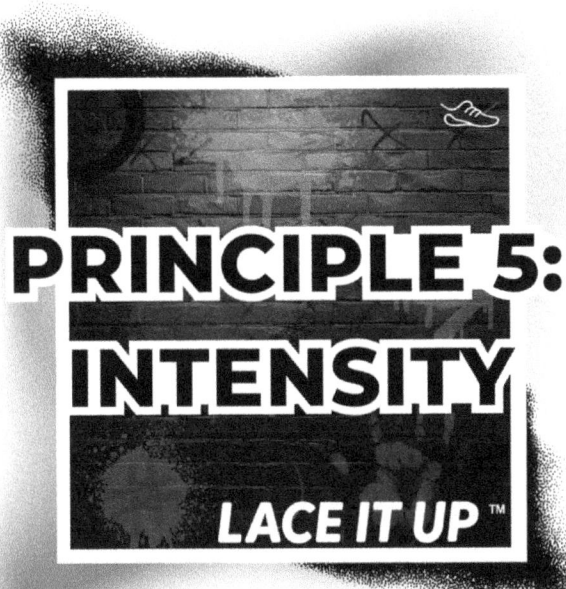

"Intensity refers almost exclusively to the human will and the ability to command your muscles to contract against the only real resistance—your own mind."

– Mike Mentzer

Principle 5: Intensity

Fact: to be successful in team sports, intensity isn't an option. It's the line between being present and being unstoppable. It rushes in at the critical moment, the buzzer-beater, the penalty kick, the unbreakable defense when every second counts. Can you feel the pulse? Intensity is how you move, how you breathe, how your mind becomes razor-sharp and every distraction disappears.

The world slows down for most. For you, intensity speeds everything up. The field shrinks, voices blur, time distorts. There's a singular mission, a play, a possession, a ball, a block. There is no tomorrow. Every muscle is tight, every thought is singular, execution is a must. Nerves become fuel and you charge into the moment. Intensity rips away excuses. It's the storm, the surge, the challenge staring directly back at you as the clock ticks down.

Focus on these seconds because they matter. In intensity's glare, hesitation dies, doubts disappear, and everything irrelevant gets shut out. You listen for the right sound, the coach's call, the sharp scrape of cleats, the snap of a pass, and you launch. Intensity isn't chaos. It's clarity carved by urgency. The ordinary becomes electric. The next play is everything.

Consider what intensity asks of you. It's full focus, speed, and urgency. It's every sprint run as if you're being chased. It's every cover with eyes wide; every rep finished with nothing left in the tank. The greatest players aren't casual. When intensity is demanded, they give it. Period. No compromise, no apology, no fear.

You either burn for this moment, or you get burned by it. You don't coast, you don't hope it works out, you make it happen. Now. Intensity separates wishers from doers, contenders from champions. It's not sustainable for hours. That's not what it's for. It's for critical moments, decisive strikes, and game-on demands when everything rides on what you do next.

Why write this way? To put you inside the pressure, the chase, the expectation. To let you feel the urgency in your bones, not just your mind. This opening isn't meant to comfort; it's meant to wake you up. To push past the effort of reading these words. To prepare you to respond, not someday, but now. To expose intensity as the mental weapon that flips games, careers, and lives. Do you feel it?

Intensity doesn't tolerate "kinda." It demands your whole focus, your whole fire. As you dive into this chapter, don't just read, lean in, speed up, focus, and lock in. Welcome to your intensity chapter. Let's get it.

What Intensity Looks Like

Effort and intensity are related.

Let's think of them more as cousins, and not twins.

The difference between effort and intensity:

1. Effort is the amount of work you put in.
2. Intensity is the speed, focus, and urgency of that work.

Think of it like this, jogging around the field is effort. Sprinting with your eyes locked on the ball, arms pumping, determined to get there first …that's intensity. Doing a drill half-

Principle 5: Intensity

speed just to finish is effort and attacking every rep like it's game day …that's intensity.

- ✗ Effort question: "Did I try?"
- ✓ Intensity question: "How hard and how focused was I when I tried?"

Lesson: Effort gets you on the field. Intensity sets the tone once you're there.

Analogy: The Light Bulb vs. the Laser

Picture two sources of energy: a light bulb and a laser. Both use power, but in totally different ways. A light bulb throws light everywhere, spreading energy across the whole room, turning dark into day, but never packing much punch in one spot. It's great for seeing, but not for changing anything.

Now, think about a laser. It takes that same energy, focuses it tightly on one point, and suddenly it can slice through metal, cut diamonds, and even travel for miles without fading. It doesn't just shine, it leaves a mark.

Effort is the bulb: it can light up your day. Intensity is the laser: it can change the game. Most players burn energy like a bulb, working hard, but a little scattered. Champions focus theirs. They aim their fire on the play at hand, lock in, and push their energy through the target instead of letting it leak out everywhere.

Don't just be everywhere, be focused, be effective. Turn that "on switch" into a laser beam when it counts.

Lesson: Don't just give energy, focus it. Effort lights the field, but intensity wins the tough moments.

LACE IT UP

Story: Allen Iverson's Practice

Allen Iverson was one of the most electrifying players in NBA history. He was quick, fearless, and could drop 40 points on anyone. But what else is he most famous for? A press conference where he said: "We talking about practice... not a game... practice."

Here's the deal: Iverson wasn't lazy. He gave effort, he showed up. But he didn't always bring intensity to practice. He coasted. He cut corners. His coaches and teammates got frustrated, because they knew his game-day intensity was unmatched, but it didn't always carry into practice.

It's like that kid on your team who jogs through drills, but the second the scrimmage starts, they're suddenly flying around like their hair's on fire. Iverson saved his intensity for the lights and the crowds.

It worked for him because he was ridiculously talented. But what about for most players? That approach is a disaster. If you don't bring intensity to practice, you never build the habits to play with it in games.

Lesson: Effort without intensity is like showing up to practice with your shoes untied. You're there, but you're not ready to win.

Story: Kobe Bryant's Relentless Intensity

If Iverson showed what happens when you save intensity, Kobe Bryant showed what happens when you live it.

Kobe's intensity was legendary. He treated every practice like it was Game 7 of the NBA Finals. His teammates sometimes hated it. Why? Because Kobe didn't care if you were tired, sore, or just not "feeling it." If you were on the floor with

Principle 5: Intensity

him, you had to bring intensity, or he'd expose you. That was the heart of his "Mamba Mentality."

There's a story from the Netflix Redeem Team docuseries that shows it best. During the 2008 Olympics, Kobe and Team USA were facing Spain. His Lakers teammate, Pau Gasol, played for Spain. The night before the game, Kobe told his U.S. teammates: "First play of the game, I'm running right through Pau's chest."

They laughed. Kobe and Pau were close friends. Surely, he wouldn't.

Tip-off came. First play. Spain ran exactly the set Kobe predicted. He saw Pau coming to set the screen… and he lowered his shoulder and went straight through him.

Gasol hit the floor. The U.S. bench exploded. Kobe didn't even blink.

Why? Because to Kobe, intensity meant sending a message. This wasn't Lakers practice. This was USA vs. Spain, and Kobe wanted to prove to his teammates that gold came before friendship.

Intensity doesn't just raise your game. It forces everyone around you to level up.

That's the pros. But intensity isn't just for NBA legends. I saw it firsthand in youth soccer, thanks to a coach who lived it every second, Coach Charles.

Story: Coach Charles on 11

Let me tell you about one of the earliest and most important voices in my boys' soccer journey: Coach Charles.

Coach Charles is intensity in human form. Honestly, if you looked up intensity in the dictionary, it might just say: "See Coach Charles." Practices with him weren't quiet. Games weren't calm. He was always the loudest voice on the field, and not in a bad way. His voice pulled every ounce of energy and focus out of his players.

When he praised a kid, it wasn't a polite clap. It was a roar:

"YES! THAT'S HOW WE PLAY!"

When he demanded more, it wasn't optional. It was sharp, focused, and urgent:

"SPEED!"
"PRESS!"
"BABY SHOT BRO!"

That was Coach Charles in full surround sound.

He didn't just expect intensity. He modeled it. His body language, his voice, his passion, it was always 11 on a 10 scale. And the kids? They caught it. My boys learned from him that intensity isn't just about working harder. It's about attacking every moment with urgency, focus, speed and fire.

And here's the funny part: even when Coach Charles shows up as a spectator, you still hear him. Out of nowhere, from across the field, his voice cuts through:

"LET'S GO JACK — SPEED!"

"YEAH CARSON — WHAT A SAVE!"

Nobody knows exactly where it's coming from, but everyone feels it.

We're grateful for Coach Charles because he instilled that lesson early. To this day, when my boys are dragging, I'll remind them, "Channel your inner Coach Charles." And instantly, their focus, speed, and urgency sharpen.

Lesson: Intensity is infectious. When a leader lives it out loud, the team rises with them.

Principle 5: Intensity

Why Intensity Matters

If effort gets you in the door. Intensity kicks that door off its hinges and demands a seat at the table. Feel the difference? It's the difference between just showing up and showing up ready to make a play, every single time. Intensity is where good habits become big results. It's what cranks up the pace, lifts the team, and makes your effort count for something that actually shifts the outcome.

Intensity isn't just extra energy, it's a ruthless commitment to making every moment, every rep, and every inch matter. The fastest teams play with it. The toughest players harness it. Coaches can see it, opponents can feel it, and the game always rewards it.

The qualities Intensity brings:

1. Urgency. Every play matters.
2. Focus. No wasted movements, no wasted words.
3. Fearlessness. Intense players aren't afraid to make mistakes. Their fearlessness can even intimidate opponents.
4. Energy Transfer. Intensity spreads just like effort and teammates feel it.

Lesson: Intensity makes average effort look extraordinary.

Analogy: The Volume Knob

Effort is like turning the music on. Intensity is how loud you play it. At low volume, you can hear it, but it doesn't move you. It's why we turn up the music when that song we like comes on.

At max volume, the whole room feels it. It's the same on the field. You can jog around and "play the song," but nobody feels your presence. Or you can crank it up, sprint, act fast, communicate with authority, and suddenly your intensity pulls everyone in.

Lesson: Don't just show up and play the song, turn it up so your team feels it.

Intensity: Key Takeaways

- ✓ Effort is how much you give. Intensity is how hard and how focused you give it.
- ✓ Effort is the light bulb. Intensity is the laser.
- ✓ Intensity brings urgency, focus, and fearlessness.
- ✓ Intensity is contagious — it raises the energy of the whole team.

Intensity: Reflections

1. Think of a teammate who always brings intensity. How does it affect the team?
2. When was the last time you confused effort for intensity? What was missing?
3. Which area of your game could use more intensity — conditioning, skills, or communication?
4. How do you feel when your team's intensity drops?

Intensity: Practice

Rep Check:
- ✓ In your next drill, ask yourself, "Am I going through the motions, or am I attacking this like Kobe would?"

Game Speed Rule:
- ✓ Do one part of practice at full game speed. Then expand it each week.

Intensity Buddy:
- ✓ Pair with a teammate and hold each other accountable for energy level in practice.

Laser Drill:
- ✓ Pick one focus (like first touch or communication) and attack it with laser-like intensity all week.

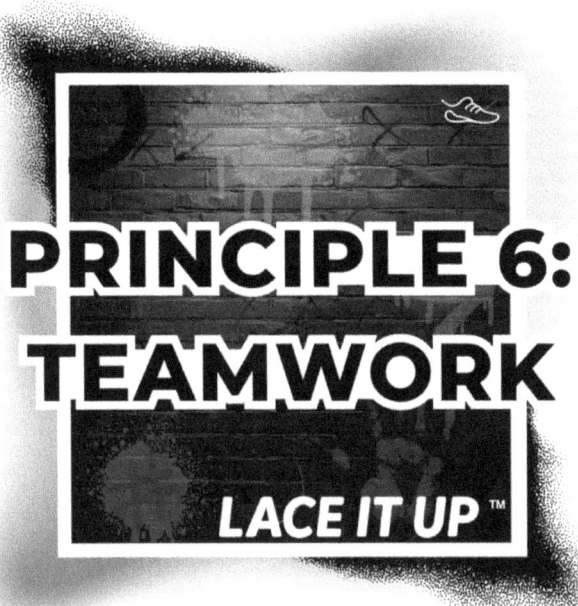

PRINCIPLE 6: TEAMWORK

LACE IT UP™

"The strength of the team is each individual member. The strength of each member is the team."

– Phil Jackson

Principle 6: Teamwork

No one makes history alone. The highlight reels, the buzzer-beaters, or the clutch moments, just look closer and you'll see a cast of teammates moving together, and amplifying each other's strengths. Anyone can celebrate the superstar, but champions know teamwork is what turns noise into harmony and solo brilliance into something legendary.

Teamwork starts with a choice. Will you play for stats or for the people beside you? Every winning team in sports history, whether it's the Patriots in Super Bowl LI, the Golden State Warriors during their dynasty run, or a high school squad defying expectations, they prove it's not just about talent. It's about how those talents fuse into one powerful, resilient unit.

Imagine a team on game day. The crowd gets loud, expectations get heavy. The star player has the spotlight, but the outcome depends on every member—starters, subs, role players, and those cheering from the sidelines. The best teams play like a chain, each link working together, each member pulling their weight. You feel it in the extra pass, the quick cover, the pride that comes from lifting up others, and in the actions that define champions, no matter what the scoreboard says.

Let this chapter challenge your habits. Teamwork is passing when you could shoot, celebrating the assist, covering for a tired teammate, and owning your unique role. Coaches talk about "buy-in," but real buy-in is showing up for the hard conversations, supporting others when it costs you minutes, and giving the game your heart no matter what the box score says.

Now, pause. Great teams don't play as a collection of individual stars; they move as one. Not just in sport, but in life as a whole. Even in workplaces, classrooms, or families, those who elevate everyone around them make the biggest impact.

What Teamwork Looks Like

Nobody lifts a trophy alone. Teamwork is the superglue of every championship story, holding talent and heart together. One superstar without a team is like noise with no melody. But when every player shows up for each other? That's a full orchestra, making music you'll remember.

Teamwork stands out in the little things and the big moments. You see it every time a pass goes to the open teammate instead of forcing a wild shot just for the glory. You see it when someone sprints back on defense to cover a tired teammate, or when the bench goes wild for an assist that mattered as much as a goal. Real teams notice effort, not just points. They recognize the players who play their roles with pride, owning every block, screen, cover, and hustle play—even when the spotlight misses them.

Teamwork looks like this:
1. Making the smart pass, not the selfish shot.
2. Setting your ego aside to cover for others, even if it means more work and less credit.
3. Lifting each other up, whether that's celebrating an assist, a block, a sacrifice bunt, or a winning penalty save.

4. Wearing your role with pride, knowing a great team needs more than stars—it needs glue guys, defenders, communicators, and leaders in every spot.

Lesson: Great teams don't play with multiple individual players. They play as one.

Analogy: The Puzzle

A puzzle looks impossible when it's just loose pieces scattered on the table. Some pieces are bright and obvious, some are dark corners you barely notice, but every single one is essential. Miss just one? The image is forever incomplete.

Teamwork works exactly the same way. In soccer, you need the attacking spark up front, the engines in midfield, the sturdy defenders, and the fearless keeper, with all starters and role players making the picture work. Move to basketball, and you'll find centers, forwards, guards. Some are there to score, some to lock down defense, some to dish out assists or grab rebounds, but every player owns a piece of the team's identity. Switch to football, and suddenly every position is its own shape—quarterbacks, linemen, receivers, backs, special teams. Track and field? Every relay, every event, every handoff matters. Baseball and softball rotate through hitters, pitchers, catchers, utility players—nobody does it alone. Do you see where I'm going here?

The uniforms, the plays, the trophies might look different, but in every sport the principle holds firm: Your piece, your role, matters. No one wins if the "corner piece" doesn't lock in. No championship is built if the "edge" doesn't form its line. The flashiest scorer or the highlight-reel play only happens because every other piece fulfilled its job.

So, whether you're blocking a shot in volleyball, setting a perfect screen in basketball, covering your zone in hockey, or cheering like crazy from the dugout, you're completing the picture. Without you, the story has a hole in it. Every. Teammate. Matters.

Lesson: Don't wish for someone else's piece. Focus on making yours fit perfectly. That's how winning teams, across every sport, bring the whole puzzle together.

Story: The Greatest Super Bowl Comeback

In 2017, the Atlanta Falcons had the New England Patriots right where they wanted them. Super Bowl LI. Halftime. Falcons up 21–3. Then they scored again in the third quarter, 28–3.

Game over, right?

I remember sitting at home in Atlanta, watching Falcons fans who were ready to pop champagne and celebrate a big Super Bowl win. And as a Giants fan, I'll be honest, part of me thought this was finally Atlanta's chance to join the club. My Giants had beaten Tom Brady in two Super Bowls, and it looked like the Falcons were about to earn their own badge of honor: "We've got Brady's number too."

But Tom Brady had other plans.

What happened next wasn't about one superstar saving the day. It was about a team that refused to quit and trusted each other every single play. The Patriots' defense tightened up. The offensive line gave Tom Brady the time he needed. Receivers ran crisp routes. Running backs fought for extra yards. And then came that catch, Julian Edelman, surrounded by three Falcons players, reaching out with fingertips to snag the ball inches from the turf. You could feel the shock on every Falcons fan's face in Atlanta and around the country. The power of teamwork gave the Patriots new life.

Principle 6: Teamwork

Bit by bit, stop by stop, catch by catch, the Patriots clawed back. And with every play, their belief in each other grew. Brady's leadership mattered, sure. But without the offensive line holding blocks, without receivers making circus catches, without the defense buying them one more possession, the comeback doesn't happen.

By the time the Patriots tied the game at 28–28 and forced overtime, you could feel the momentum shift like a tidal wave. The Falcons were stunned. The Patriots were locked in. One overtime drive later, it was over. Patriots 34, Falcons 28. The biggest comeback in Super Bowl history.

For Falcons fans in Atlanta, it was heartbreak. For me as a Giants fan, it stung a little too because instead of the Falcons stealing Brady's crown, he reminded us all why he's called the GOAT (Greatest of All Time).

The Patriots' comeback wasn't magic. It was an entire team pulling the rope in the same direction, refusing to let go.

Lesson: Teamwork isn't flashy. It's trust. It's grit. It's doing your job on every play so the teammate next to you can do theirs.

Story: Carson the 5-Star Teammate

My son Carson has always been a standout soccer player. Confident, skilled, gritty, and intense. But basketball? That was a different story.

When he tried out for the 6th grade middle school basketball team, he wasn't the most polished player on the court. He could hustle, sure, he could defend, yes, but he wasn't putting up any highlight reels. Making the team was both challenging and humbling because unlike soccer, where Carson was often 'the guy', here he was just trying to keep up.

LACE IT UP

What got him a spot wasn't his jump shot or ability to drive to the basket. In my opinion it was his ability to be a 5-star teammate. Let's unpack that together.

Carson understood something that most middle school athletes don't: you don't need to be the star to make a difference. He embraced being the ultimate teammate. He looked for the open pass. He cheered for his teammates from the bench. He was first to high-five, first to celebrate a bucket, and always the loudest voice encouraging the team.

Here's the kicker: he didn't get much playing time. And that can crush a middle schooler's spirit. I'd be lying if I said it didn't bother Carson, nobody wants to sit. But Carson and I had some deep conversations about it. I told him, "Playing time isn't in your control. But being a 5-star teammate is. Coaches and players notice effort, energy, and encouragement, even if you never touch the ball. Just because you're not the best scorer doesn't mean you can't be the best teammate." And he believed it. He bought into it. His perspective shifted.

At times, it felt like he was the team mascot, always fired up, always supporting, always pushing the group forward. But in practice, he worked just as hard as anyone. He learned the drills, ran them clean, asked questions, and set the tone for intensity. He made the team better whether or not he played a minute on gameday.

One night, I saw just how much his teammates valued him. The game was tight, playoffs on the line. Carson hadn't played a single minute, and the star player, the one who usually had the spotlight, came out for a quick rest. He grabbed a drink, nudged the coach and said, "put Carson in."

That moment hit me hard and touched my heart. The star of the team wanted my son in the game, not because of points or rebounds, but because of who he was as a teammate.

Principle 6: Teamwork

Full disclosure, Carson didn't go in. The stakes were too high, and the coach needed his best five on the floor. But that didn't take away from the impact he made. He didn't show up on anyone's box score that night, yet he helped his team in more ways than he'll ever know.

Teamwork is about what you give to the group, not what you get from it. Carson showed me that sometimes the greatest players on a team don't always directly influence the scoreboard but they show up in the spirit of their teammates.

Lesson: You don't need game minutes to make a difference.

Analogy: The Chain

Picture a heavy chain pulled taut, every link locking in, holding the full weight of the load. That's a team. Tough, steady, built to bear the pressure of the biggest moments. Can you picture it? But what if there's one weak link? That's all it takes for everything to snap.

On every team, every player is a link. Football needs linemen just as much as quarterbacks. Baseball demands focus from the ninth hitter as much as the cleanup slugger. In hockey, it's not just the goal scorers, it's the grinders and the defenders keeping the ice safe. No one gets a pass. If one person cheats a drill, skips extra work, plays lazy on a possession, the entire chain suffers. You can feel it. Mistakes get magnified, trust erodes, and the whole team buckles under pressure.

But when each link is strong—when every teammate brings focus, hunger, and accountability—the chain gets unbreakable. Suddenly, the impossible task becomes light work. The defining challenges of the season get met, lifted, carried together.

LACE IT UP

The best teams obsess over their link. They strengthen it daily, knowing that greatness is never about just one superstar. It's about everyone refusing to let the chain break on their watch.

If you want a team that can carry anything, from setbacks to championships, you owe it to yourself and your teammates to make your link the strongest it can be. Teamwork demands it, and so does the scoreboard.

Lesson: Teamwork means strengthening your link so the whole team holds strong.

Why Teamwork Matters

1. Connection. Teammates play harder when they trust each other.
2. Resilience. Teams that pull together bounce back from setbacks.
3. Accountability. Everyone pushes each other to stay sharp.
4. Joy. Winning is fun, but winning together is unforgettable.

Lesson: Teams win trophies. Lone wolves don't.

Teamwork: Key Takeaways

- ✓ Teamwork is the glue that makes talent stick.
- ✓ Every role matters — big or small.
- ✓ Unselfish play creates unstoppable teams.
- ✓ Your success is tied to the people next to you.

Teamwork: Reflections

1. Who on your team makes others better? What do they do?
2. When was the last time you put the team's needs above your own?
3. Do you celebrate teammates' successes as much as your own?
4. How do you react when your team struggles? Do you lean in or pullback?

Teamwork: Practice

Assist First Drill:
- ✓ In your next game, look for one chance to set up a teammate instead of taking the shot yourself.

Cover Move:
- ✓ Pick one practice to focus on covering for others, tracking back when a teammate is beat or filling in their space.

Teammate Spotlight:
- ✓ Give a shoutout to someone on your team who doesn't usually get credit. Later, think about how it made you and them feel.

Chain Check:
- ✓ After practice, rate your "link" on a scale of 1–5. Did you strengthen or weaken the chain today? Think about ways to strengthen the chain.

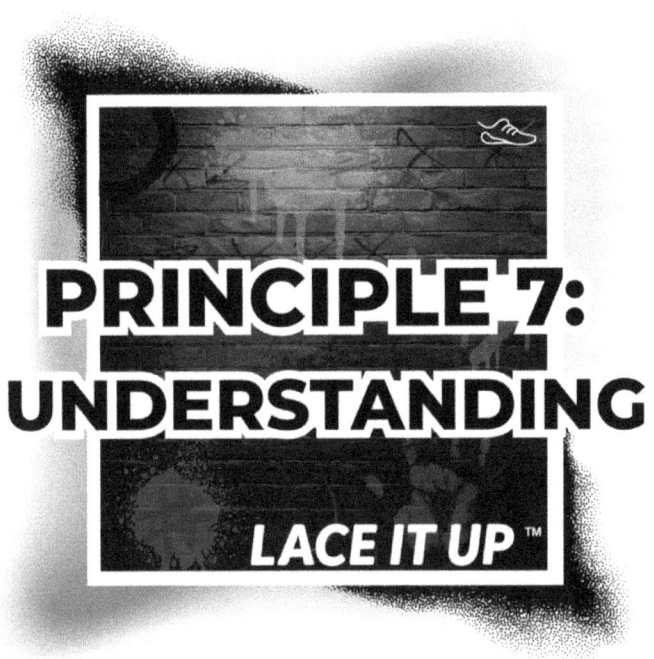

"It's what you learn after you think you know it all that really counts."

– John Wooden

Principle 7:

Understanding

Understanding is an athlete's greatest edge. Talent puts you on the field. Effort and intensity keep you in the game. But it's understanding, developing real game IQ, the drive to learn, the itch to know "why?", that separates the player who barely survives from the one who thrives. Understanding is what every champion, coach, and "next-level" athlete obsesses about.

A lot of players search for shortcuts in the weight room or on the track. Every athlete, from rookies to All-Pros, knows you have to build your body if you want a shot. But the game changes for the players who build their mind just as fiercely. The smart ones never stop asking questions, taking notes, watching film, breaking down mistakes, and chasing the answer behind the answer.

Curiosity wins. The player who leans in, gets honest about weaknesses, dives into extra scouting, and hunts for patterns rises the fastest. Talent fades, legs tire, luck bounces the other direction. But understanding, the habit of learning, is always there to light the way. It's the force that helps players make the split-second read, the calm decision under pressure, the perfect pass that only comes because they've studied what no one else bothered to see.

LACE IT UP

The best athletes and most successful people are lifelong learners. They close gaps by asking the right questions, solve problems by reviewing and adjusting, and squeeze every drop of value from practice by understanding both what to do and why it matters. Every post-practice note, every journal entry, every "What went wrong?" and "How do I fix it?" stacks up over time. Learning isn't just about knowledge; it's about adaptation. Small improvements, made consistently, become unstoppable advantages.

If you've ever wondered why some players always seem a step ahead, reading the play, beating opponents to the ball, seeing passing lanes first, isn't luck. They've built their minds with the same sweat, reps, and discipline that go into their bodies. Champions make curiosity a habit and aren't embarrassed to be "caught" learning. They embrace it as a super power. They know every lineup, every moment in film study, every mistake in practice can teach them something new.

Why does this matter? Because games aren't won by athleticism alone. They're won by players who react just a little bit faster, who can adapt on the fly, who see danger before it's obvious. Understanding isn't just for the "coach's favorite player" or the straight-A student. It's a skill, built through effort, repetition, and a willingness to turn every experience, good or bad, into wisdom.

So, what should you do? Be relentless in pursuit of the "why." Write down what you see and feel. Ask questions and act on the answers. Take pride in studying the game, yourself, your teammates, and even your opponents. Make your journal as beat-up as your shoes. Celebrate little "Aha!" moments as much as big wins.

Just like reps make muscles grow, honest reflection and constant analysis through thinking and writing make your mindset powerful. Your curiosity is your ticket to a smarter,

Principle 7: Understanding

more adaptable, more complete version of yourself, on the field and in life. Build it, flex it, use it. Understanding is your edge.

Understanding: The Strongest Muscle You Have

Everyone talks about grit and heart. Coaches yell about effort. Trainers obsess over reps in the gym. All of that matters, but understanding is what sets apart the elite from the average. Most athletes do the work to build their body. Very few do the work to build their mind. That's your secret advantage.

Understanding starts with curiosity. The best players are the ones who never stop asking: "Why did that work?" "Why did that fail?" They want to know what's under the hood. To dominate in sports, you need more than fast feet or strong arms. You need to read patterns, anticipate the next play, sniff out weaknesses, and pass that intelligence to your teammates. It's like being a coach while you're still in uniform.

If you're already putting in the hours on skill drills, film, and workouts, here's your next challenge: put the same energy into learning the game inside and out. Be the one who remembers details others forget. Study your mistakes without fear. Notice the subtle hints, who's tired, where the space is, what the other team wants. Ask smart questions and actually use the answers. Make every practice a lesson, not just a grind.

You don't have to be the smartest person in the room. You just have to be relentless about learning more and getting better. Write down lessons, track your goals and setbacks, and look for patterns after every drill. Over time, those habits aren't homework; they are cheat codes. And who doesn't love a good cheat code? To this day I remember the cheat code that gave me unlimited lives for the game Contra, on the original Nintendo Entertainment System (up up, down, down, left, right, left, right, B, A, select, start). Cheat codes like this help you play faster and smarter, with more confidence and less panic.

LACE IT UP

Here's the truth: no one remembers the player who ignores their weaknesses or makes excuses for mistakes. Everyone remembers the one who wants to know why the play broke, who talks through a new approach, who adapts quicker than the rest. Curiosity drives improvement. Without it, you get stuck. With it, you become the kind of teammate and leader coaches build rosters around.

In this chapter, you'll see how understanding powers every part of the journey: learning from games, from friends, from failure, and from yourself. It's preparation, it's reflection, it's the edge that lets you make the better decision a step before everyone else, whether it's a key play or a clutch choice off the field.

So don't just work hard. Work smart. Build your "why" muscle every day and let curiosity fuel your climb. Give your mind the same respect you give your body. Your understanding is what holds it all together, and in the long run, it's what sets you apart.

What Understanding Looks Like

Understanding is about seeing the bigger picture, connecting the dots, and playing three moves ahead. The best players aren't just fast; they're smart. They know the "why" behind every "what" and turn that knowledge into better choices, quicker reactions, and smarter plays.

Game IQ isn't memorizing a playbook, it's living it. It's the curiosity that fuels your questions in film study, the awareness that shows up in the clutch, and the edge that makes the difference between just being there and being unstoppable.

Understanding looks like this:
- ✓ You know your role and how it helps the team win.

Principle 7: Understanding

- ✓ You read score, time, momentum, and matchups.
- ✓ You anticipate what opponents want and take it away.
- ✓ You study teammates so you can feed their strengths.
- ✓ You learn rules and avoid careless mistakes.
- ✓ You ask good questions and apply the answers.

Lesson: Effort moves you. Intensity speeds you up. Understanding points you in the right direction.

Story: Jackson and the Seven-Touch Challenge

A perfect day at the park. Just me and Jackson getting touches. He ran his warm up, hit a few drills, and pushed a couple of weak spots. Low pressure. High bonding. After about 90 minutes he was packing up.

I said, "I have a fun challenge." I described a seven-touch juggle: left foot, right foot, left thigh, right thigh, left shoulder, right shoulder, head, then receive clean on the foot. He laughed. "No way. I can't do that."

I had seen a young player do it online, but I kept that to myself. Some kids can be funny about that. Instead, I raised the stakes. "You get 30 minutes. If you complete it, we stop for ice cream. If you do not, you tried and practiced something new. Deal."

He locked in. Feet and thighs were fine. The shoulders were the problem. He almost never uses his shoulders like that. Fail. Adjust. Fail. Adjust. Fail. Each miss dialed up his focus. "How much time left." Twenty-five. Then twenty. He stopped trying the full sequence and isolated the shoulder-to-shoulder exchange. Reps. Reps. Reps. He found the rhythm, popped to the head, cushioned the final touch down to his foot, and stuck the landing with 18 minutes on the clock.

We celebrated like we won the lottery. Some people gave strange looks but we didn't care.

Then I surprised him. "You have 12 minutes left to prove it was not luck. Do it again." The smile dipped for a second. Then he said, "Bet." Ice cream was already secured, but pride was on the line. With two minutes left, he nailed it again. Second celebration, even louder.

That is understanding. Break the problem into parts. Get curious. Adjust. Test. Repeat.

Lesson: Skill grows when curiosity meets a clear plan.

Story: Derek Jeter's Flip and the Power of Preparation

October 13, 2001. Yankees at A's. American League Division Series. Game 3 in Oakland. The Yankees were down two games to none and clinging to a 1–0 lead. Seventh inning. A shot into the right field corner. The throw home sails up the first base line. The runner is flying toward the plate. It looks like an easy score.

Then Derek Jeter appears in a spot you would not expect a shortstop to be. He sprints across the diamond, intercepts the off-line throw, and makes a backhand shovel flip to the catcher, who tags the runner out at the last possible second.

People called it instinct. It was. It was also understanding. The Yankees had scouted that stadium and that play. Jeter knew an off-line throw might drift up the line, and he knew exactly where to be to save it. That flip was study, positioning, anticipation, and trust in a plan.

The Yankees won the game and then the series. One moment of understanding kept the season alive.

Principle 7: Understanding

Lesson: Preparation turns information into advantage. Understanding puts you in the right place before everyone else arrives.

Understanding Yourself

Why understanding yourself matters

Most youth athletes do not want to write. It feels like homework. Again, writing is a cheat code for learning. When you write, you slow your brain just enough to think clearly, you remember more, and you spot patterns faster. Pros do it because it works.[6]

On HBO's Hard Knocks, I watched a Buffalo Bills player pull out a beat-up notebook to write and review notes and goals. He said it was something he did every day. That is not an accident. That is how you get better on purpose.

What writing does for athletes

1. Locks in memory. Notes stick. You recall them in games.
2. Builds self-awareness. You find what helps and what does not.
3. Shrinks mistakes. You turn "I messed up" into "Next time I will do ___."
4. Fuels motivation. Small wins stack up.
5. Creates a plan. You do not just try harder. You try smarter.

LACE IT UP Success Journal, Your Writing Edge

Don't let journaling be something the pros do, make it your own built-in advantage. When you take a few minutes to write each day, you're not just reflecting, you're actually building the habits, mindset, and accountability that separate good from great. You dial in your focus, see your progress add up, and learn something new about yourself with every entry.

That's why I built a LACE IT UP Success Journal to accompany this book. Want to put all of this into action? It isn't a journal for perfect handwriting or long essays. It's designed to be short, direct, and actually get used, day after day. You'll track your wins, challenges, micro-goals, and the little habits that add up to big results and much more. It's a mirror for your progress, a launchpad for the next step, and a blueprint for building success on purpose.

Journaling is Journaling

You don't have to use the LACE IT UP Success Journal to get the benefits of writing. Any notebook, phone app, or scrap of paper works if you actually use it. The real magic comes from showing up, not from what your journal looks like. Consistency beats style. Two minutes beats zero. Short and honest beats perfect and polished, every single time.

That said, I designed the LACE IT UP Success Journal to make things simple, focused, and actionable (because keeping all your wins, development areas, habits, and goals in one spot makes it more likely you'll stick with it). But if you prefer your own method, here's a game plan you can use anywhere:

Daily (about 2–5 minutes)

Wins (1): One thing you did well today and why it worked.

Challenges (1): One thing that needs work and what caused it.

Micro-goal (1): One specific action for tomorrow.

Energy Stars (1–5): How you showed up today.

Mindset Note (1 line): Add "yet", turn a struggle into a not-yet moment.

Weekly Summary: 3–2–1 + 1

    3 Wins from the week.

    2 ACGs (Areas for Continued Growth).

    1 Plan for when you'll work those ACGs next week.

    +1 Gratitude for someone you appreciate and why.

Lesson: The method matters less than the habit. Show up for yourself on the page, and your progress on the field will follow.

LACE IT UP

Example of a Daily Entry

Wins: Timed press twice and won the ball. Anticipated the pass early.

Challenges: First touch on switch balls floated. Misjudged flight.

Micro-goal: Ten passes off the wall tomorrow.

Energy Stars: 4 of 5

Mindset: Heading accuracy is not there yet.

Example of a Weekly Summary

3 Wins:

1. First touch cleaner in tight space.
2. Communicated early on set pieces.
3. Better recovery runs after turnovers.

2 ACGs:

1. Back post awareness.
2. Driven passing technique.

1 Plan:

- ✓ Tuesday and Thursday after practice, 15 minutes of back post reps. Saturday morning, 50 driven passes.

+1 Gratitude:

- ✓ Coach T for the guidance and praise during my last bicycle kick attempt. Helped me build the confidence to keep trying them.

"I hate writing" options

Not everyone loves to write. That's normal. What matters is the reflection, not the grammar. Here are some low-pressure ways to stick with your journaling habit:

- ✓ Try bullet points only. Skip long sentences. Just write a few quick hits: what worked, what didn't, what to try next.
- ✓ Use voice to text. Record a 30-second voice memo after practice or a game, then jot down three quick bullets from what you said.
- ✓ Set a timer for 60 seconds, challenge yourself to blitz through the page. No rewrites, no overthinking.
- ✓ If you're stuck, start with "Today was…" and finish the sentence. Or just rate your day 1–5 with a single reason why.
- ✓ Remember, it's your journal. One line or even a single word is better than skipping it. Aim for consistency, not perfection.

Pro Tip: Go for maximum results, minimum stress. The point isn't fancy writing; it's better thinking and better habit development.

Make it stick

- ✓ Same time, same place. Tie it to dinner or bedtime.
- ✓ Keep it visible. Notebook lives with cleats or water bottle.
- ✓ Set a timer. Begin.
- ✓ Accountability buddy. Choose someone to help you be consistent.

LACE IT UP

Sleep: the silent superpower

Sleep is not extra. It is part of training. Understanding the power of good sleep separate the good from the great. Most teens do best around 8 to 10 hours a night, and school-age kids need even more.[7] Good sleep improves reaction time, focus, mood, and decision-making.[8,9] Translation for game day: faster reads, cleaner touches, better choices.

Simple sleep playbook

1. Keep the same schedule, if possible, your body loves rhythm.
2. Screens off about 60 minutes before bed. Put the phone to bed before you.
3. Keep the room cool, dark, and quiet. Think cave, not carnival.
4. Short naps are fine if needed, about 10 to 30 minutes, early afternoons when possible (especially on weekends).
5. On big tournament weekends, protect the two nights before.

Pro Tip: If late homework and early practice are squeezing sleep, talk to a parent or coach. Lack of sleep is a performance issue, not a toughness test.

Lesson: Sleep is how your body and brain cash in your practice.

Fuel: Simple Nutrition and Hydration

Let's keep it real: everyone's nutrition needs are different, and no, I'm not a registered dietitian. Use common sense, respect allergies and family choices, and talk with a pro if you need a real plan. But here's the lesson I try to pass on to my kids and

Principle 7: Understanding athletes: what you eat is more than a treat, it's fuel for performance. Every bite, every sip, is either powering your battery or draining it.

You've probably heard the classic line, "It doesn't have to taste good to be good for you." There's some truth there (though good food can actually taste great!). The important part is shifting your mindset: don't just think about what you crave, think about what's going to help you run farther, recover faster, and hit your next goal. Food isn't just about taste, it's about what will fuel you best for the next big play.

So next time you grab a snack or plan a meal, ask: Is this giving me what my body needs, or just a quick sugar fix? Treat what you eat and drink as your on-field advantage. Your future self and your game will thank you.

The Performance Plate

Match your plate to your training day. On hard days, include more carbs for fuel. On easier days, lean a little more on veggies and protein.[10] Always aim for:[11]

- ✓ Carbs for energy: rice, pasta, potatoes, oats, fruit, whole grains
- ✓ Protein for repair: chicken, fish, eggs, yogurt, beans, tofu
- ✓ Color for health: vegetables and fruit
- ✓ Fluids: water first, sports drink only for long, hot, or very intense sessions[12]

Timing you can trust[13]

- ✓ 3 to 4 hours before: a carb-centered meal with some protein.

- ✓ 60 to 90 minutes before: a light snack you know sits well, like a banana with yogurt or half a peanut-butter sandwich.

- ✓ During: sip regularly. Water for practices under an hour, consider electrolytes for heat or long events.

- ✓ After: grab a quick carb plus protein to refuel, then eat a full meal within a couple of hours.

- ✓ Tournament tip: Pack familiar snacks. Between games, keep food simple and light. Save heavy meals for the end of the day.

Lesson: Food is fuel, hydration is wiring. Get both right and your work shows up.

Understanding Others

You can't win big if you only know yourself. Great teams, and the best athletes, are experts at reading the people around them. They know that every player, coach, and opponent has strengths, quirks, and patterns that can be learned, and leveraged. Champions don't just react; they anticipate. They notice who leads, who needs a nudge, who cracks under pressure, and who brings the heat when it matters most.

The more tuned in you are to your teammates, the more you make everyone better, including yourself. The more you scout your competition, the more you turn matchups into mismatches on purpose.

Understanding others is part detective work, part leadership, and all about leveling up your team IQ. Study people as closely as you study plays. That's how you become a trusted teammate, a difference-maker, and the kind of player every coach wants on the field.

Principle 7: Understanding

Teammate Scouting

If you're not using the LACE IT UP Success Journal, keep scouting notes on your teammates. One page per teammate. Update over time.

Name / Date / Position

Strengths: Where do they shine?

What motivates them: What lights them up?

ACG: What is one observed area for continued growth?

How can I help them: How can you help them continue to grow?

Notes from Games/Practices: Write down general notes and observations.

Example of a Teammate Scouting Page

Date: Sept 10 **Name:** Francis R. **Position:** Winger

Strengths:

- ✓ Explosive first step, receives well to feet, strong back post runs.

What motivates them:

- ✓ Shoutouts, quick eye contact, clear targets.

ACG:

- ✓ Checks out after a turnover. Needs a "next play" cue.

How can I help them:

- ✓ Practice saying "good effort, next play".

Notes from Games/Practices:

- ✓ Starts with energy and pace, loses steam about halfway through.

Study the Competition

Foundational questions to guide your eyes in any sport:

1. Key threats: Who can beat you if ignored. Strong foot or go-to move.

   ✓ Tendencies: Where they build and how they like to attack.

2. Pressure points: What breaks under stress. First touch, set pieces, transitions.

3. Space map: Which zones they leave open and how often.

4. Patterns after turnovers: Do they rush and force it, or regroup and recycle.

5. Emotional swings: Do they lose focus after a bad call or late in games.

Write one strength to respect and one weakness to attack. Keep it simple. Use it.

Lesson: Understanding others turns you into the kind of teammate and competitor coaches' trust.

Understanding the Game

Knowing the game isn't about having the quickest feet, it's about having the quickest mind. The best players aren't always the fastest runners; they're the fastest thinkers. They can read what's coming, spot space before it opens, and get where they need to be, before everyone else even sees it. That's what "being a student of the game" really means.

Game intelligence is built, not born. It comes from watching with intent, asking "why" after every play, and turning film or practice into a study session. If you want to level up from good to game-changer, start by sharpening your mental playbook every time you watch, coach, or compete.

Principle 7: Understanding

Watch like a data analyst

You want to play smarter? Start by watching smarter. Don't just zone out or follow the ball, watch games the way top coaches and pros do, looking for the patterns that decide wins and losses. Here's a simple way to analyze film: Grab your notebook, set up three columns, and let's go to work.

Look beyond the highlight reel. Ask: What's actually working? What keeps breaking down? What's the real reason behind each moment, good or bad? Every shift, every sequence, has a cause.

Use this simple structure the next time you watch, whether it's film, live games, or even your own practices:

- ✓ **Working:** What is creating chances or stops.
- ✓ **Not Working:** What keeps breaking down.
- ✓ **Why:** Your best read on the cause.

The Three-Moment Read

This is the lens to analyze any clip or live sequence.

1. Before: Where is the space? Who is unmarked? Who is tiring?
2. Trigger: What starts the action? A press, a run, or a specific pass.
3. After: What should the next action be? Did they choose it?

Applying Understanding in Leadership

Understanding powers leadership because it shapes how you think, not just how you act.

LACE IT UP

Tips for success:

- ✓ Add "yet." "I cannot do this yet" tells your brain to keep learning.
- ✓ Praise the process. Effort, strategy, and improvement matter.
- ✓ Treat mistakes as data. Not shame. Data. Adjust and try again.
- ✓ Set process goals.

Leader phrases that build understanding

"Tell me what you are seeing."

"Here is the plan. Any gaps."

"Try this, then we will evaluate."

"Good idea. Let us test it for five minutes."

Teach back leadership

If you can teach a concept in 30 seconds, you truly understand it. Make teammates your classroom. One tip. One rep. One improvement.

Lesson: Leaders learn in public and invite others to learn with them.

Translating Understanding Beyond Sports

Understanding is not only for the field.

School

- ✓ Before homework, write the learning goal at the top. Example: "I can solve two-step equations."
- ✓ After homework, write one sentence. "What clicked and why."

Friends and Family

- ✓ Ask clarifying questions before reacting.
  "What did you mean by that?"

- ✓ State needs clearly.
  "I need five quiet minutes, then I am all yours."

Life Logistics

- ✓ Learn one new skill a month. Cooking a simple meal. Budgeting your allowance. Time blocking a busy day.

- ✓ Build a checklist you can reuse. Pack list. Morning routine. Tournament day gear.

Lesson: Understanding is a life skill. Use it everywhere.

Why Understanding Matters

Understanding:

1. Speeds decisions so you play fast and think calm.

2. Reduces mistakes through better positioning.

3. Builds trust because you see what others see.

4. Saves energy by putting you in the right place early.

5. Keeps you safe by reading risky moments before they explode.

Understanding: Key Takeaways

- ✓ Know yourself. Track Wins, Challenges, and Micro-goals.

- ✓ Know your body. Protect sleep and fuel on purpose.

- ✓ Know others. Learn how teammates and coaches think and play.

LACE IT UP

- ✓ Know the game. Watch like an analyst and look for patterns.
- ✓ Lead with a growth mindset. Add "yet," praise the process, use teach backs.
- ✓ Take it beyond sports. Understanding makes life smoother.

Understanding: Reflections

1. What is one strength you can lean on this week, and one ACG you will develop?
2. Which teammate do you understand best? What do you do that helps them shine?
3. When you watch games, what patterns do you notice first? Why those?
4. Where could a simple "yet" change how you feel about a challenge?
5. How many hours did you sleep the last two nights, and did you feel the difference?
6. What did you eat and drink before your last game, and how did you feel in the first ten minutes?

Principle 7: Understanding

Understanding: Practice

Success Journal, 2-5 Minutes:
- ✓ Write Daily
- ✓ Write a Weekly Summary, 3–2–1 + 1

Teammate Scouting:
- ✓ One page per teammate. Strengths, Motivation, ACG

Data Analyst Watch:
- ✓ Fill Working, Not Working, and Why

21 Day Understanding Challenge

Build the habit. Test the value. Decide for yourself.

Days 1 to 21: Do the work
- ✓ Do your Success Journal every day. 2-5 minutes. Bullets are fine.
- ✓ Do your Weekly Summary 3–2–1 + 1 at the end of each week.
- ✓ Protect sleep and fuel with the simple checklists.

Day 22: Honest analysis (Answer in writing):
- ✓ Did this help me understand myself better? Can I name clear wins, ACGs, micro-goals, and how sleep and fuel affected me?
- ✓ How did this help me understand others better?
- ✓ How did this help me understand the game better?

If you saw improvement, keep going. You found a tool that works. If it didn't help you improve, adjust or drop it. Your time matters.

LACE IT UP

Mindset Tip: Habits feel awkward before they feel helpful. Give it the full 21 days. Then choose with a clear head.

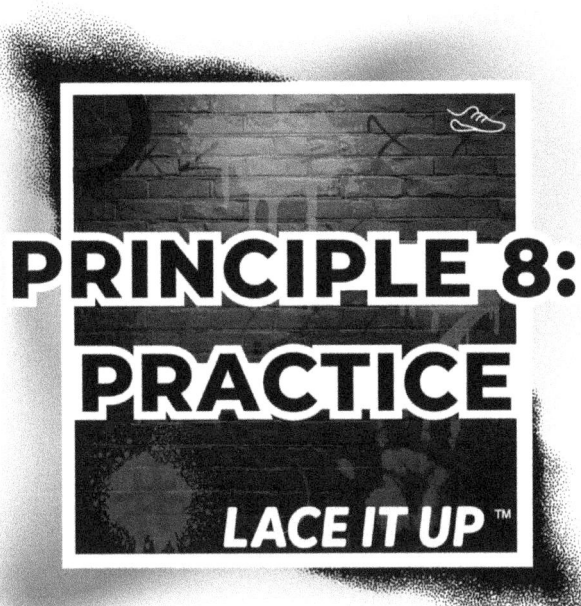

"Amateurs practice until they get it right. Professionals practice until they cannot get it wrong."

– Unknown

Principle 8: Practice

What do you really want as an athlete? Chances are, you want confidence—the kind you can count on when the score is close, the stands are full, and your heart is pounding. Most people think confidence comes from being the most talented. Here's the truth: real confidence comes from all the quiet hours you put in when nobody is watching. The secret is practice, not magic.

Some athletes believe practice is just about showing up, getting sweaty, and checking off drills. But just moving does not equal improving. Champions do more than chase sweat; they chase skills they can trust when pressure is highest. There's a serious difference between working hard and actually getting better. Want to know the difference? Purpose.

Training with purpose means way more than "just get better." It means every rep, every drill, every adjustment is connected to something specific you want to improve. You are not out here collecting hours for bragging rights. You are sharpening skills that will show up when it matters—under the lights, with eyes on you, and pressure on 10.

Don't just count the number of shots, passes, runs, or blocks you do. Start counting how many you did with intention. This world is full of athletes who say they "work hard." The ones who rise above are the ones who make every session count. They treat skill like a muscle. It grows when you train it on purpose. Practice is your workshop.

Effort with purpose builds the edge nobody sees. Study the best pros, college stars, or even outstanding players on your own team. What sets them apart isn't luck or hype. It's the quiet reps done on purpose. It's repeating the same drill until it seems boring, then dialing in and sharpening every detail. It's not skipping over mistakes; it's fixing them and owning every adjustment that makes the next rep better.

Everyone wishes for huge games and big wins. It's rare to hear someone wish for more practice. But that's exactly where trust is built. Trust in your touch, your read, and your routine. When the big moment shows up, so does all the intentional work you invested in practice. This chapter is your blueprint for practice that means something. Not perfect, but always purposeful.

What Practice Looks Like

Remember, practice is not just showing up, it's training with purpose. The goal is not sweat for sweat's sake. The goal is to build skill you can trust under pressure.

Good practice looks like this:
- ✓ You start with a clear target, not "get better."
- ✓ You work at the edge of your ability, not the middle.
- ✓ You chase quality reps, not just more reps.
- ✓ You build both sides of your game, strong foot/hand and weak foot/hand.
- ✓ You get feedback and adjust quickly.
- ✓ You end with a note about what to try next time.

Principle 8: Practice

Lesson: Practice makes permanent. Only perfect practice makes progress.

Story: Stephen Curry's Quiet Reps

Everyone sees the logo threes on TV. Not everyone sees the routine that makes them possible.

Before games, Steph moves like a metronome. Two-ball dribbling to wake up his hands. Eyes up. Shoulders quiet. Then form shots from close range. He is not trying to look cool. He is checking alignment. Feet set. Elbow in. Follow through. Net whisper.

He backs up a step. Repeat. Back up again. Repeat. He flows into catch and shoot, then off the dribble, then side steps. The pace never rushes. If a miss sneaks in, he does not act surprised. He resets his feet, breathes, and runs the same motion again like a scientist rerunning an experiment.

Kids crowd the sideline to watch, phones out, whispering about the tunnel shot. Steph smiles sometimes, but the routine does not change for the crowd. It would look the same in an empty gym. That is the point. He is not practicing for applause. He is practicing for trust. So that when the fourth quarter is loud and his legs feel heavy, his body remembers what his mind almost forgot.

There is nothing flashy about quiet reps. They are simple. They are steady. They are the reason the big moments feel normal. When you see the celebration after a deep three, remember what happened an hour earlier. The quiet reps built the loud moment.

Lesson: Practice is not a performance. It is a promise you make to yourself so the big shot feels like just another rep.

Story: The Wiffle Ball Reactor Drill

As a keeper, your hands are your everything. Reaction time. Hand-eye coordination. Clean catches. In our backyard, Carson and I built those skills with tennis balls. I tossed two at a time and he snapped them back in rhythm, left then right, like juggling without the drop. We laughed when I sped it up and he still kept beat. It was fun, but it was also pressure.

After a big win, a teammate's dad came over to congratulate Carson. He had recently retired from the NFL as a wide receiver. When he talks hands, you listen. He said, "Try wiffle balls." Those holes make the flight unpredictable, he explained. If you can read and catch that, a soccer ball will start to feel slow.

So, we bought a bag of wiffle balls and I grabbed my pickleball paddle. Summer evenings turned into rapid fire sessions. Pop. Pop. Pop. Some balls knuckled, some tailed, some died early. Carson learned to read the wobble, move his feet first, then meet the ball with soft hands. When the pattern got messy, we laughed, reset, and kept going. We were not chasing perfect. We were training calm in chaos.

A month later, a deflected shot dipped late in a match. Old Carson might have been surprised. New Carson lifted, caught, and rolled the ball out like it was routine. The work showed up.

Lesson: Make practice harder than the game. If you can catch a bad wiffle ball off a pickleball paddle, a clean strike on Saturday feels simple.

Why Practice Matters

If you want real confidence on game day, you have to build it before the crowd shows up. You can't fake trust in your game. You have to earn it when no one is watching. Practice is more

Principle 8: Practice

than showing up and working hard. It is where you separate yourself from the athletes who are just busy from the ones who actually get better. Here are the benefits to investing time in practicing:

1. Confidence: Practice gives you proof you can do it.
2. Consistency: Reps turn good days into most days.
3. Speed: Clean technique makes decisions faster.
4. Trust: Coaches play athletes they can predict.
5. Durability: Good mechanics protect your body.

The Practice Recipe

Random training does not build reliable skills. Great training is like a recipe you can follow on any day, in any sport. Use this five-step system to make every session count:

1. Target: Name a single skill in one sentence.
   For example: "Driven pass off the ground, 20 yards."
2. Design: Pick a drill that focuses only on that skill.
   "Wall work with markers at ankle height."
3. Standard: Set a clear number, time, or goal.
   "30 attempts, 20 clean strikes."
4. Feedback: Decide right away how you will know if you improved.
   "Ball stays below shin, hits tape. If not, adjust plant foot."
5. Review: Write one line in your journal about what worked and what needs fixing.
   "18 of 30 clean. Plant foot crept back. Fix tomorrow."

Here is the secret: being clear on what you are working on is always better than just working until you are tired.

LACE IT UP

Lesson: Clarity beats intensity when it comes to getting better.

Block, Random, and Game-speed

If you want to build skills that actually show up in games, you need three types of practice:

- ✓ Block practice: Same skill, same spot. Builds form.
  Example: 50 passes to the same target.

- ✓ Random practice: Same skill, different looks. Builds adaptability.
  Example: Vary distance, angle, first touch.

- ✓ Game-speed practice: Add pressure and decisions. Builds transfer.
  Example: First touch, scan, pass while a partner closes you down.

Work through them in that order. Form first. Flex second. Fire last. Mastering this recipe will help you build skills that stand up under pressure and show up when you need them most.

The 20-Minute Personal Session

No field? No court? No problem. You do not need fancy gear or a huge space. You just need a ball, your focus, and twenty minutes.

- ✓ Minutes 0–5: Touch circuit. Inside, outside, taps.

- ✓ Minutes 5–10: Weak hand or foot only. Passing or finishing pattern you can repeat.

- ✓ Minutes 10–15: Decision drill. Receive, scan, play to a moving target.

- ✓ Minutes 15–20: Finisher. Ten perfect reps of your priority skill. If a rep is sloppy, do it again.

Principle 8: Practice

End with one line in your journal and a star rating for focus.

Common Practice Traps (and quick fixes)

Even the hardest workers can get stuck making the same practice mistakes. It is easy to fall into old habits, take shortcuts, or repeat what feels comfortable instead of what actually helps you grow. Smart athletes do not just train hard. Smart athletes train with awareness and adjust when things are off. Before you hit the field, court, or gym, know the most common practice traps and be ready with quick fixes to avoid them. Turning these little mistakes around will make every session matter a whole lot more.

- ✖ Mindless reps: You are moving, not improving.
  - ○ **Fix:** Say your target out loud before each set.
- ✖ Highlight chasing: Only practicing what you already do well.
  - ○ **Fix**: Start with your ACG first, then earn your favorite drill.
- ✖ Line hiding: Standing at the back of the drill line.
  - ○ **Fix:** Volunteer to go first.
- ✖ No feedback: You can't tell if you improved.
  - ○ **Fix:** Use tape, cones, a basket, or a friend to keep score.
- ✖ All gas, no form: You train fast and reinforce bad habits.
  - ○ **Fix:** Slow down until the technique is clean, then add speed.

Analogy: The Pencil

Practice is like sharpening a pencil. A dull pencil can still write, but the words come out messy. Lines smudge, letters wobble, and you spend more time fixing mistakes than making progress. Try playing your best game with a dull pencil—that's like showing up without practicing. It just won't look or feel right.

Sharpening the pencil means putting in the work. It means those extra reps, the focused drills, and the patience to get better when nobody's watching. When your pencil is sharp, your writing is clear, your moves are crisp, and your confidence shows.

Don't skip the sharpening step. Don't grab a dull pencil and hope for magic. Be the player who puts in the effort to sharpen every day. The best stories and the best games start with a sharp pencil.

Lesson: If you want clean work on game day, sharpen in practice.

Practice with Patience

Practice with patience is one of the hardest things for any athlete. Watching highlight reels online can make you feel behind, like everyone else is perfect and never makes mistakes. That feeling is normal, but it does not reflect the truth. Remember that what you're seeing is likely the best of what that person can do. What you're not seeing are the countless mistakes and setbacks that led to the highlight. Progress does not happen overnight. The skills you see on game day are built through slow, steady effort, and lots of ordinary, boring reps when nobody is watching.

When you start to feel frustrated that you are not improving fast enough, remember that patience is a skill too. It takes practice to stay focused and keep showing up when results do not come quickly. Every athlete who has made it to the top has spent months or even years stuck in the middle, working on the basics and trusting that their effort would pay off in the end.

Sticking with your routine, celebrating small steps, and relying on your journal to spot growth will help keep you level during the slow stretches. Use tough days and setbacks as a signal to pause, reflect, and check in with your coach or teammates. Skill built slowly is stronger and lasts longer. Patience will help you get there.

Tips for Practicing Patience

- ✓ Write down progress, even if it feels small.
- ✓ Notice what you learned, not just what went right.
- ✓ Trust your routine even when results are slow.
- ✓ Avoid comparing yourself to highlight reels. Focus on your journey.
- ✓ Use setbacks as feedback, not as failure.
- ✓ Talk to a coach or teammate when you feel discouraged.
- ✓ Remind yourself that skill built slowly lasts the longest.

Lesson: Practicing patience keeps you steady during the ups and downs.

Practice With People

Practicing with others is one of the most powerful ways to improve your game. When you practice alone, you get better, but practicing with teammates pushes you to a whole new level. It builds communication, trust, and timing. You learn how to read each other and play as a unit. This is where skills turn into teamwork and effort turns into momentum. The habits you build here set the foundation for success on the field. Let's break down what it really means to practice with people and how to make every session count.

- ✓ With a coach: Ask for one cue. "What is the one thing to fix today."
- ✓ With a teammate: Trade reps. One works; one watches and gives feedback.
- ✓ With a parent: Use them as a clock, a passer, or a scoreboard. Thank them.

Practice When You Are Not 100 Percent

We all have days when we are not feeling one hundred percent. Maybe you are tired, sore, or just not quite right. The way you show up on those days matters. Skipping practice is the easy choice but falling behind is not an option if you want to improve.

That said, if you are truly sick, the right move is to stay home and listen to the advice of health professionals about when you can safely return to practice. Showing up even when you do not feel your best but are well enough to be there is what separates players who make excuses from players who make progress. Here are some ways to get the most out of practice when you are not at your peak.

- ✓ Watch your position only and track spacing.
- ✓ Do band work or balance work if cleared.
- ✓ Journal three notes you learned from the sideline.

Lesson: There is always something you can train, even if it is your mind.

Tie It Back to Your Journal

Your success journal is your secret weapon for getting better. After every practice, take a few minutes to write down what worked and what needs work. When you put your thoughts on paper, you lock in the lesson. You can see progress over time, spot patterns, and set clear goals for your next session. Writing in your journal keeps you honest and focused. It turns practice from just showing up into a real step forward. Use your journal to capture your wins, your struggles, and your plan to improve. This simple habit will help you get sharper, stronger, and ready for whatever comes next.

As a reminder, here is the format shared in the prior chapter:

- ✓ One win: what felt better and why.
- ✓ One ACG: what still needs attention.
- ✓ One micro-goal: what you will do tomorrow.
- ✓ Energy Stars: rate your energy level.

Small words now save big mistakes later.

Practice: Key Takeaways

- ✓ Clear focus beats mindless movement. Know exactly what skill you are working on before each drill.
- ✓ Practice with purpose by aiming for quality reps, not just quantity.
- ✓ Use practice time to build habits that hold up under pressure. Consistency beats last-minute effort.
- ✓ Push yourself to practice with teammates and learn from each other. Teamwork in practice creates trust for games.
- ✓ Show up even on days when you are not feeling 100 percent, but know when to rest if you are truly sick.
- ✓ Keep your success journal close. Write what you learn, what you improve, and what your next step is after every session.
- ✓ Avoid common traps like chasing favorites or practicing without feedback. Stay aware and adjust to keep improving.

Practice: Reflections

1. What skill would change your game the most if it improved this month?
2. Do you practice your strengths more than your ACGs? Why?
3. Where in your sessions do you usually lose focus. What will you change?
4. Who can give you quick feedback this week?
5. How will you know practice is working? Name your proof.

Practice: Practice

Two Cue Rule:
- ✓ Pick two form cues and say them before every set.

Weak Hand or Foot Window:
- ✓ Five minutes a day on your weak side for 21 days.

Laundry Basket Target:
- ✓ Build a home target and track makes.

Volunteer First:
- ✓ Be first in two drills every practice this week.

Game-speed Finisher:
- ✓ End each session with five perfect, fast reps.

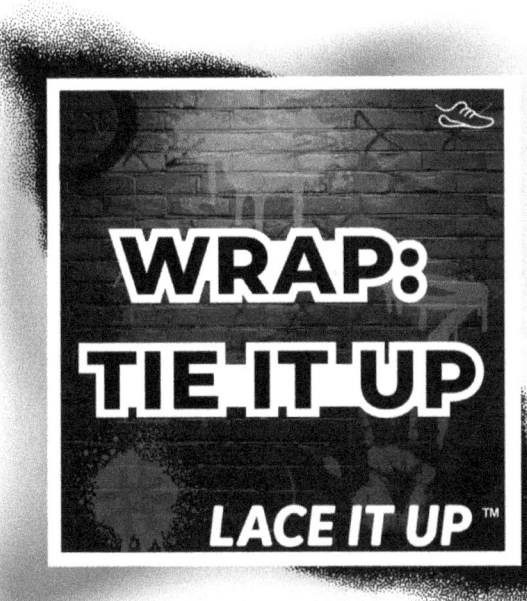

"Start where you are. Use what you have. Do what you can."

– Arthur Ashe

Wrap: Tie It Up

A new journey starts today

There is a reason we end the same way we began. You bend down; you lace up. Simple act. Big meaning. Every time you tie your laces, you choose to show up. That choice is the quiet start to every great story.

You just worked through eight principles. Leadership, Attitude, Communication, Effort, Intensity, Teamwork, Understanding, and Practice. Maybe a few came naturally. Maybe a few stretched you. Good. Growth usually lives right outside of the edge of comfort. Keep going.

Here is what I hope you carry with you. You do not need an appointed title to lead. You do not need perfect conditions to bring a strong attitude and a growth mindset. You do not need a microphone to communicate clearly. You do not need an audience to give honest effort. You do not need a packed stadium to play with intensity. You do not need to be the star to be a five-star teammate. You do not need a genius brain to build understanding. You do not need fancy gear to practice with purpose. You need a decision. You need a plan. You need the courage to repeat it.

If we met on the sideline today, I would tell you this. I believe in the power of small, steady habits. I believe in people who make hard things simpler. I believe in youth athletes who treat others with respect when the whistle goes against them. I believe you can be that person. Not someday. Now. I believe in you.

What matters most going forward

- ✓ Keep your standard. Be the example that sets the tone. Even on tired days.
- ✓ Keep your signal strong. Your attitude is Wi Fi for your team. Make it a connection, not static.
- ✓ Keep the talk clear. Short cues. Early cues. Listen as much as you speak.
- ✓ Keep doing the work. Effort does not need attention to be real.
- ✓ Keep the volume with purpose. Intensity should lift the team, not drain it.
- ✓ Keep playing for each other. 'We' beats 'me'. Always.
- ✓ Keep learning. Yourself, others, and the game. Curiosity and being a lifelong learner is your advantage.
- ✓ Keep sharpening. Practice is where you write the habits you want the lights to reveal.

You will not be perfect. Neither am I. We are perfectly imperfect in the pursuit of excellence. There will be days the pass goes long, the shot sails high, the ball gets past you, the sub comes earlier than you want. There will be days when your Energy Stars are two out of five. Write the journal entry anyway. Own it. Adjust it. Try again tomorrow. That is how real progress is made.

The 'Pass It On' Challenge

You have learned a lot here. Skills, drills, habits, and a new way to see the game. The real test is what you do with it. Do not stash it away or keep it for yourself. The fastest way to grow as a leader and as a teammate is to give your knowledge away.

Teach one tool you picked up to someone younger. Show a little brother or sister how to log a win in their journal, or help a friend cue up the right thought before a drill. Share a phrase that helped you stay positive or locked in. A good word travels, and you never know how much someone might need it.

Step up and lead a drill at practice. Are you nervous? Good. That is the whole point. That's where growth comes from. You will learn more by teaching others than from any workout you do alone. If you see a teammate struggling, offer a tip or encourage them to keep going. Build the kind of team you would want to play for.

Passing it on does not just help your teammates—it makes you sharper, too. When you make an effort to teach or explain, you have to slow down and truly understand the skill. That kind of learning lasts. At the same time, you help lift the whole group higher. Teams where athletes share knowledge are always tougher and tighter.

Here is your challenge. In the next week, teach, share, or lead. Pick one tool, one habit, or one pep talk and give it away. Start a ripple and watch it grow. When you pass it on, you become the teammate everyone remembers. Be the kind athlete who makes the whole team better.

LACE IT UP

Your next week, simple and clear

Tonight:
- ✓ Write one page in your Success Journal. One Win, one Challenge, one micro goal, Energy Stars, one line with "yet."

Tomorrow:
- ✓ Give three purposeful shoutouts. One for direction, one for encouragement, one for awareness.

This week:
- ✓ Be first in line for two drills. Start with your ACG before your favorite skill.

Next 21 days:
- ✓ Choose one habit from this book. Track it daily. On day 22, evaluate with honesty. Keep it if it works. Adjust if it does not.

Thank your people

No one gets here alone. Every athlete, even the pros you watch on TV, has a story full of the people who helped them along the way. You do not have to look far to find yours. Think about the coach who called you out when you needed to hear the truth, the teammate who stayed after practice to run sprints with you when you were struggling, or the parent who sat in the car with you after a tough game, listening and reminding you that you are more than a score.

Gratitude makes you stronger. It is not just about saying thanks to be polite. It is about honoring the effort other people put in so you could succeed. Every late-night ride, every cheer from the stands, every packed snack, and pep talk at breakfast built your foundation. When you thank your people, you show that you see their sacrifice. You recognize what it takes to push you forward.

Do not just think it, say it out loud. Tell your coach, "Thanks for being hard on me. I know you care." High five the teammate who picked you up when you lost your spark. Give your parents a real thank you, no eye roll, just for all the little things they do. Write it in a note, send a text, or share it in the group chat.

Gratitude is a team skill. When you say thank you, you bring the team closer. You let people know you are paying attention, that you value what they bring and who they are. It builds trust. It builds bonds. The simple act of giving credit makes the whole group stronger. Teams that share gratitude play harder for each other and enjoy every win more.

Make it a habit. Thank your people after every game, each practice, or every long drive. Start and end the season with appreciation and spread it around like confetti. It feels good. It lifts the group. It keeps you humble. And someday, somebody will thank you. Pass it on.

A Final Word for Young Athletes

Let's be honest. The world loves medals, trophies, and highlight reels. Some people will measure you by what hangs on your wall or gets posted online. That is not how I measure you. The truth is, I care more about the kind of person you are becoming than any hardware you could stack up. I hope you see the value in becoming someone who is dependable, honest, and willing to work hard when nobody else is watching.

You are going to have moments that feel amazing. Big wins, loud celebrations, and days when your skill catches you

LACE IT UP

by surprise. Enjoy those. You earned them. But here is something nobody tells you when you first tie up a pair of laces. You will also have tough days. You will lose games you thought you should win, watch somebody else make the play you dreamed about, and wonder if you belong. Every athlete faces these moments. They hurt, but they help you grow. Losing does not mean you are broken. It means you are getting strong.

Take pride in your habits. The way you show up matters more than the score at the end. Laugh with your teammates, share the hard work, and keep the game fun even when practice gets boring. The best teammates help each other get better. Find ways to make the field, the court, or the locker room a better place every time you leave. That is a win for everyone.

Character gets practiced every day. Be the athlete who shakes hands after a loss and congratulates the player who made a great play. Cheer hard for your teammates and own your mistakes. Nobody needs you to be perfect. We need you to keep going, to learn from tough days, and to push yourself and the team forward. That is what makes you strong. That is what success looks like for life, not just sports.

Do not forget the habits you built in this book. The drills, the journal entries, the routines you practiced when nobody was watching—those are your tools for the future. Winning feels good but a strong heart and steady mind feel better. When you hit a setback, remember every late-night practice and every early morning workout. Trust the quiet work you did. That kind of effort tells the real story.

Here you are, laces ready. Heart steady. Mind clear. You know what matters now: the eight principles, your plan for tomorrow, and the plan for next week. Tie them up for real and take the next step. Go live what you have learned. You have got what it takes to become the kind of athlete (and person) you are proud of. Make mistakes. Learn from them. Help your teammates. Leave the field a little better than when you arrived.

That is how champions are made. Not just from winning, but from the way you play, the way you practice, and how you show up for others. Now get out there. Remember the lessons, the laughs, the losses, and the victories. Show everyone what "LACE IT UP" really means.

Final Word for Parents and Coaches

Thanks for showing up. It is not easy hauling kids to early morning games, remembering their cleats, their water, and sometimes even their sense of humor. I have worn every hat in the youth sports world: parent, coach, ref, team manager and chief snack hauler. If you have ever sprinted back to the house because someone forgot essential gear, you are one of us.

Your presence matters. Kids play better, learn more, and have more fun when the adults around them are calm, clear, and caring. Even if the coffee is cold and the grass is wet, you set the temperature for the team. The loudest cheers and the softest advice both mean more than you know.

Lead with positivity. Celebrate effort, not just winning. I'm not saying go out and produce "participation trophies", let me be clear. If your kid manages to make it to practice with matching socks a smile, and a positive outlook, that is worth a fist bump. Mistakes are part of the game and a big part of growing up. When something goes sideways, treat it as what it is—a chance to learn. Say, "You are still learning, take it in and adjust for next time" instead of turning it into drama. Bonus points if you manage this without sighing or waving your arms like a third base coach. It's easier said than done—I get it!

Model what truly matters. Our kids copy what we do. They hear the words we use with coaches, refs, and other parents. Some days you will be cool as a cucumber. Other days you

LACE IT UP

might want to yell into your hat or drop kick your pillow. Show respect no matter how wild the game gets. Years from now, what you did will matter more than what you said.

For parents, fight the urge to coach from the sideline—think of it as letting your athlete drive the bus. Yelling, "Get back on defense!" or "Use your left!" rarely helps in the heat of the moment and usually distracts the player. Instead, trust the coaches, enjoy the ride, and remember you do your best work in the car on the way home because empathy and ongoing support is where you can shine bright light a diamond.

Build strong relationships. Youth sports are as much about high fives as high scores. Help your kid learn every teammate's name, toss compliments around, and keep the group texts positive. A goofy nickname or post-practice snack run might be what your player remembers. My wife and I have issued nicknames like "Jack-Attack," and "Flying Squirrel," and my kids have slung them back like "Papa burro" (translated: 'daddy donkey' because I'm always hauling things around for the family) and "Big Sus" (because sometimes you'll find me secluded on a sideline with the hoodie and sun glasses on, quietly evaluating game play). Sports can also be about team-building disguised as fun.

Draw a hard line against bullying, both on and off the field. Leaders stand up for what's right and build safe environments for every kid. If you hear something out of line, step in and make it clear that your team will not play that way. It matters more than any tactical advice.

Keep car rides short and sweet. If you want a magic formula, try this:

"I love watching you play."

"What did you learn today?"

Wrap: Tie It Up

"What is one thing you want to work on next week?"

If you need an advanced move, throw in, "should we stop for a snack?" That alone may turn the whole day around.

Protect the fun. Sports are supposed to be joyful. Effort follows excitement, and growth follows effort. If the game starts feeling like homework or too much pressure, pause and help your player reconnect to the joy. That joy is the reason kids stay in the game year after year. If you are chasing wins and missing joy, slow down and look for what made the game special in the first place.

Coaches, hats off to everyone who rallied the troops, untangled the drills, and made time for every player. You make sport a safe place for kids to grow. Thank you for clear plans, honest feedback, and for calling timeout when needed for both the team and the parents.

Parents, thank you for jumping into the mess with both feet, finding lost uniforms, and cheering even when the game is about mud, not medals. You protect the joy and help build character, commitment, and community.

Here is your challenge. Be the positive force in the room, on the field, and in the group text. Help every kid feel seen and valued, even when they miss the big shot. Check in with your coach, offer a "You did great," and mean it. Turn every "oh no" into "now we know." Give yourself credit for hard days and keep moving forward. Youth sports need grown-ups who show up, mess up, bounce back, and try again. Let your actions be the story kids remember.

Here's a true pro-tip for every parent on the sideline: cheer just as loud for your child's teammates as you do for your own kid. Kids always recognize their parents' voices and expect to hear encouragement from them, but something powerful happens when another parent shouts their name in celebration or appreciation. When a young athlete hears a teammate's parent notice their hustle, attitude, or great play, their face lights up. It fills them with pride, fuels their effort, and gives them an extra reason to keep pushing.

If every adult in the stands made it their mission to celebrate all the kids, not just their own, you would see the energy and confidence on your team skyrocket. Try it this season. You never know which word of encouragement is going to be the one that sticks with a player long after the final whistle. Show kids that the whole team matters, and watch what happens next.

If we can work together—to cheer, encourage, listen, and laugh—we will build teams that last and form players who become great people. After all, nobody ever won a championship alone. Let's give our young athletes every reason to keep tying their laces and chasing the next adventure.

Lastly, give yourself some grace. Yes, being an athlete is tough, but let's be real: it's not always easy being the parent or coach either. We are all making big sacrifices to help kids chase their dreams, and some days you may only have half a tank left after a long, stressful day. Mix in kids going through their own emotional rollercoasters, and showing up with a smile is not always a walk in the park. Trust me, I get it—I live it right beside you.

Take a few deep breaths and remember your why. Find your meaning, your reason, the bigger picture that keeps you coming back. We are lucky to be in this struggle with our kids, even when it's hard. There are so many alternatives we would never wish for. Some days, you give what you have left and that is enough. Make sure to give yourself permission to recharge, too. If you ever see me reclining my seat in the car and catching

Wrap: Tie It Up

a 20-minute nap during practice, just know you're in good company. We all need a little rest sometimes—so we can show up strong the next time.

Tie it up. Let's play. And never forget, you are making a difference, one car ride, one practice, and one word of encouragement at a time.

Acknowledgements

This book came together the long way: steady reps, honest feedback, and many hands.

First, to my wife, Adele: thank you for your patience, honesty, and partnership through countless weekends on the sideline. You managed the load of schedules and logistics while I chased a big idea one keystroke at a time. All the while, you led a high-performance team at work, tackled the demands of a challenging career, and pursued your higher education goals—often at the same time. I am in awe of how much you take on, and inspired by the way you make it look so easy. You are the true model of "Effort" and the poster child for getting things done without excuses.

You were my soundboard in the early days, helping shape what would become these principles. You played the devil's advocate when ideas needed stress-testing, and were my biggest supporter when I needed encouragement or battled imposter syndrome. This book, and everything it stands for, would not exist without you.

To my sons, Carson and Jackson: you are my favorite teammates. Your effort, courage, and humor show up on these pages. I admire your fearlessness and your big hearts—especially the way you love your mom and our dogs. I learn more from watching you than you know. I am lucky to be your dad.

LACE IT UP

To my daughter, Marisa: I got early practice as a young father building my knowledge and experience with what would eventually become these principles during your formative years. Becoming a father at a young age forced me to quickly develop leadership skills to support a family. You were the first to teach me resilience, patience, kindness and the importance of showing up every day. Those lessons are laced into this book.

To all the coaches who shaped our family's journey, thank you for modeling intensity, care, and clarity. A special thank you to Coach Charles. You poured so much into the boys during their intro into club soccer and became a friend. You raised the standard, made the work fun, and helped them think bigger and believe in themselves.

To the parents and players in our club community: you brought the stories to life. Help with rides to practice, weather delays, tough losses, big wins—thank you for the support, lessons, laughs, and the shared experiences.

To early readers and loved ones who gave feedback: you sharpened the ideas and protected the voice. Any line that hits home probably started with your nudge.

To my mentors and colleagues: leading teams over the course of my professional career has taught me as much about sports as sports taught me about work. Thank you for the trust and the reps.

To the Bronx, where I learned grit and intensity, and to the Southeast, where I learned soccer and raised children: both are home. Both shaped this book.

And to every young athlete and family reading this: thank you for giving these pages a shot. I hope they help you lace it up with purpose, play with joy, and unlock your best self on and off the field. Go get it.

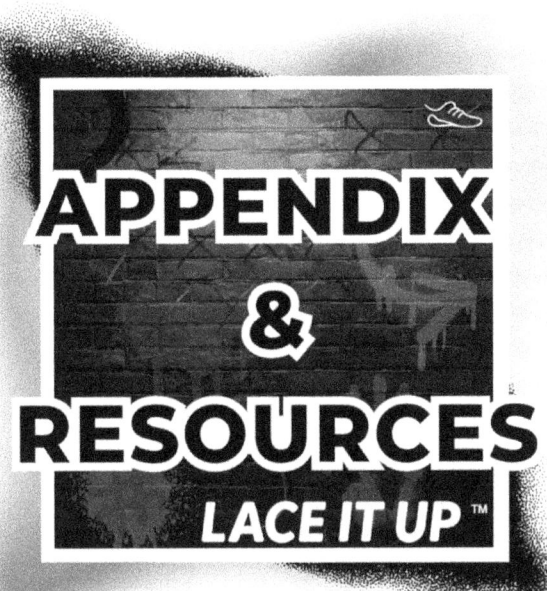

Appendix & Resources

Stay Connected with Team LACE IT UP

The journey does not stop when you finish this book. Want to keep building your skills, grow as a teammate, and stay fired up with new ideas? Visit teamlaceitup.com for resources made just for youth athletes, coaches, and parents.

Discover more about the Success Journal, designed to help you track wins, set goals, and chase progress even after the last page. You can get your own journal, dive into sample prompts, and find tips for making the most out of every practice and game.

Share your journey with us by submitting a quote after you finish the book. Your words and ideas help inspire the next group of athletes coming up. Want to bring the LACE IT UP principles to your school, club, or team? Book a speaking session or hands-on workshop. Whether you need a pep talk, practical drills, or guidance for coaches and parents, we have you covered.

Stay connected with new challenges, updates, and community shoutouts by following @teamlaceitup on Instagram. You will find stories from athletes just like you, examples of real journal pages, and strategies to keep your mindset sharp.

The LACE IT UP team wants every athlete, parent, and coach to be part of this movement. Visit teamlaceitup.com,

LACE IT UP

join the conversation, and build confidence step by step. Tie it up. Take action. See how far you can go.

Want a shortcut? Scan and connect.

You can scan the QR codes below with your phone's camera to join the LACE IT UP community online.

To visit our website for journals, updates, and resources, scan the code below:

To see our latest news, tips, and athlete stories on Instagram, scan the code below:

Just open your camera app, point it at the QR code, and tap the link that pops up. That is it. You are one click away from more ways to grow, connect, and get inspired.

About the Author

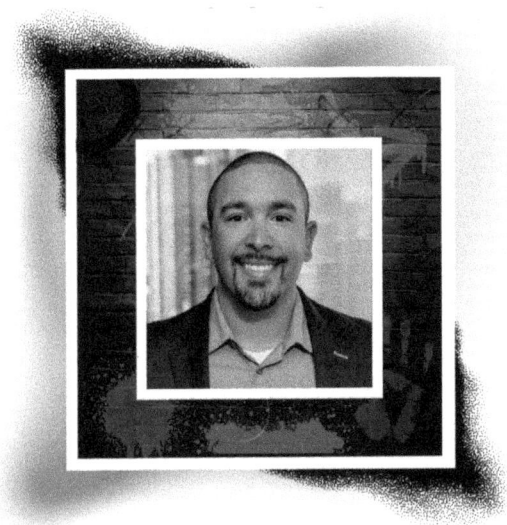

Gabriel Crespo is a dad, husband, mentor, leader and working professional. He grew up in the Bronx, New York, where structure and sport helped him steer clear of trouble, and moved to the Southeast in '99. These days you will find him and his wife Adele on a sideline with chairs, and water bottles, learning right alongside their sons. He believes great teammates are built, not born, and that small habits done with care turn into big wins over time. LACE IT UP brings together lessons from experience, family, friends, mentors, coaches, research, continuous learning and leadership at work to help youth athletes grow on the field and off it.

Eight Principles.

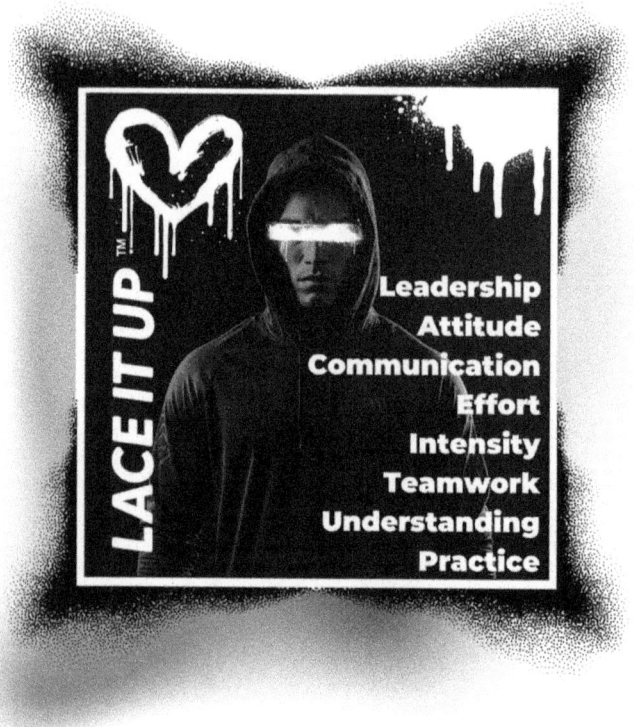

Notes

1 Burns, J. M. (1978). Leadership. New York: Harper & Row.

2 Greenleaf, R. K. (1970). The Servant as Leader. Indianapolis: Greenleaf Center.

3 Doran, G. T. (1981). There's a S.M.A.R.T. way to write management's goals and objectives. Management Review, 70(11), 35–36.

4 Dweck, C. S. (2006). Mindset: The new psychology of success. Random House.

5 Brownell, J. (2012). Listening: Attitudes, Principles, and Skills (5th ed.). Boston, MA: Pearson.

6 Mueller, P. A., & Oppenheimer, D. M. (2014). The pen is mightier than the keyboard: Advantages of longhand over laptop note taking. Psychological Science, 25(6), 1159–1168.

7 Paruthi, S., Brooks, L. J., D'Ambrosio, C., Hall, W. A., Kotagal, S., Lloyd, R. M., … Wise, M. S. (2016). Recommended amount of sleep for pediatric populations: A consensus statement of the American Academy of Sleep Medicine. Journal of Clinical Sleep Medicine, 12(6), 785–786. https://doi.org/10.5664/jcsm.5866

8 Fullagar, H. H. K., Skorski, S., Duffield, R., Hammes, D., Coutts, A. J., & Meyer, T. (2015). Sleep and athletic performance: The effects of sleep loss on exercise performance, and physiological and cognitive responses to exercise. Sports Medicine, 45(2), 161–186. https://doi.org/10.1007/s40279-014-0260-0

9 Killgore, W. D. S. (2010). Effects of sleep deprivation on cognition. Progress in Brain Research, 185, 105–129. https://doi.org/10.1016/B978-0-444-53702-7.00007-5

10 United States Olympic & Paralympic Committee Sports Nutrition Team. (n.d.). Athlete's plates: Easy, moderate, and hard training day meal models. Colorado Springs, CO: USOPC. Retrieved September, 2025, from: https://www.teamusa.org/nutrition/athletes-plates

11 Thomas, D. T., Erdman, K. A., & Burke, L. M. (2016). Position of the Academy of Nutrition and Dietetics, Dietitians of Canada, and the American College of Sports Medicine: Nutrition and athletic performance. Medicine & Science in Sports & Exercise, 48(3), 543–568. https://doi.org/10.1249/MSS.0000000000000852

12 Sawka, M. N., Burke, L. M., Eichner, E. R., Maughan, R. J., Montain, S. J., & Stachenfeld, N. S. (2007). American College of Sports Medicine position stand: Exercise and fluid replacement. Medicine & Science in Sports & Exercise, 39(2), 377–390. https://doi.org/10.1249/mss.0b013e31802ca597

13 Thomas, D. T., Erdman, K. A., & Burke, L. M. (2016). Medicine & Science in Sports & Exercise, 48(3), 543–568. National Collegiate Athletic Association Sport Science Institute. (n.d.). Nutrition fact sheets for student-athletes. Indianapolis, IN: NCAA. Retrieved September, 2025, from: https://www.ncaa.org/sports-science-institute/nutrition

For Miranda.
My brightest light in the darkest hours.
You've taught me more about love, courage,
and patience than anyone else ever could.
You are my miracle.

And for a physician I once loved:
What we shared was kindred—
fleeting, but eternal in its echo.

FOREWORD
BY WHITLEY STRIEBER

This deeply personal and profoundly unsettling account of Erik Nanstiel's close encounter experiences is a testament to the resilience of the human spirit in the face of the terrifying and, ultimately, the transformative.

Erik's story begins with ambiguous childhood encounters that evolve into a lifelong odyssey of abductions, medical procedures and psychological intrusions that cause the barriers between dream and reality to break down, leaving him clinging to memories that may not be memories at all, but also not dreams. They may be something else, a connection with events that happen on a shadow-line between realities that is in its essence beyond our our understanding. He describes the fear, the confusion, the struggle to reconcile the mundane routines of life with continuing and surreal invasions of his privacy and his mind with striking clarity.

What makes this book so compelling is not just the vivid details of Erik's encounters but the way he grapples with their implications. He asks the questions we would all ask—"Why me?" "What do they want?" —and seeks answers in his own psyche, in the stories of others who have walked similar paths, and in the broader mysteries of human evolution and consciousness. His journey is not just about the Greys or the implants or the procedures; it is about what it means to be human in a universe that may be far more complex—and far less private—than we ever imagined.

This is not a book for the faint of heart. It is a book for those who are willing to confront the unknown, to question the boundaries of reality, and to consider the possibility that we are not alone in this vast and mysterious universe. Erik's story is a reminder that the truth, whatever it may be, is not always easy to accept. But it is in the act of seeking it, of speaking it, and of reclaiming it that we find our power.

In these pages, Erik offers us more than a memoir; he offers us a mirror. It reflects not only his own journey but the universal human struggle to make sense of the incomprehensible, to heal from the wounds we cannot see, and to find courage in the face of the unknown. His story is a testament to the enduring strength of the human spirit—and a reminder that in a future where we must all confront this bizarre reality, we can, as he has in his private experience, find a way forward.

—Whitley Strieber
Copyright 2025, Whitley Strieber

INTRODUCTION

I didn't set out to write this book because I thought I had all the answers. I wrote it because I needed to put the pieces together—for myself, and maybe for others who've experienced something similar but never knew how to talk about it.

For most of my life, I carried a strange kind of silence. Memories that didn't behave like memories. Moments that didn't make sense. And feelings—deep, buried feelings—that whispered of things I couldn't explain. I tried to live a normal life. And for the most part, I did. But every so often, something would crack the surface. A vision, a missing moment, a presence in the room that vanished the second I woke up.

Only after a lifetime of scattered events did the pattern begin to emerge. What started as a string of personal experiences—dreams, encounters, missing time—gradually revealed itself as something much larger, far more organized, and deeply unsettling. These weren't random hallucinations. They were part of a structured phenomenon with roots not only in my own life, but in the lives of others, stretching back across generations. Including my own mother.

I'm not a scientist. I'm not a spiritual leader. I'm just someone who decided it was finally time to document what happened—not to convince anyone, but to confront the truth as I experienced it. Along the way, I began comparing my memories with the research, the case files, and the accounts of others who have walked a similar path. The more I uncovered, the more I realized: I'm not alone. And neither are you, if you've ever felt that eerie sense of being watched or changed in ways you can't fully explain.

This book is a record. It's a narrative of what I remember, what I've uncovered, and what I've come to suspect about the intelligence behind these encounters. It explores not only the events themselves but the possible motives behind them—motives that reach into questions about human evolution, consciousness, and perhaps even the nature of the soul.

I don't claim to know what the final truth is. But I do know what I saw, what I felt, and what I've come to understand.

If you're holding this book, it may be because you've had questions of your own. I don't pretend to offer closure—but perhaps something here will resonate with you. Perhaps you'll see a reflection of your own story in mine. And maybe, together, we can begin to push back the shadows, and the angst —one memory at a time.

– Erik

1

THE PAST IS PROLOGUE

I woke up in my garage.

Not in my bed or in my house, but in my cold, dimly lit garage, hovering off my feet above the concrete floor. My body was tilted forward at a slight angle, feet dangling, weightless. I couldn't move. I couldn't speak. I was too shocked to think. But I was wide awake.

The ceiling light was off, yet the space wasn't entirely dark. A bright, shimmering white light streamed through the side window, flickering slightly, as if from a moving source outside. My breath caught in my throat. Something—someone—was in there with me.

He stood before me, near the window, barely three and a half feet tall, dressed in black coveralls from neck to foot. His arms were long and thin, hanging at his sides as he gazed up at me with massive black eyes in the middle of his bulbous, ashen-grey head. His head was tilted upward toward me as he stared directly at me.

And then, clear as a chime, his voice entered my brain. "We can't allow you to remember our visit, because my superiors will know about it."

I had no time to react. No time to ask questions. My consciousness went black, like a switch had been flipped, and I woke up back in my bed as if nothing had happened. But something had happened.

That moment, and the many that came after, forced me to confront memories I had buried for years. Mere whispers from the dark corners of decades past. And it brought into sharp relief memories that my mother had once dismissed 67 years earlier. It was all about to come together and demand a reckoning. What I thought I knew about my life and my world view was about to change.

Who in the World Am I?

> *"Who in the world am I? Ah, that's the great puzzle."* — Lewis Carroll, Alice's Adventures in Wonderland

My name is Erik Nanstiel. I'm a graphic designer and art director by trade, as well as a single father and guardian to a nonverbal adult daughter with autism. Until a few years ago, when my daughter moved into a group home that cares for adults like her, I had been a single parent for sixteen years. My life revolved around the routines of raising a special needs child, doing everything I could to earn a living, and ensuring we had a stable home. Post-divorce, life was often a struggle—juggling bills, navigating inadequate childcare, and confronting an income that never quite stretched far enough. Throughout those years, I battled depression while striving to keep my daughter healthy and happy. When I finally "graduated" to the title of 'empty nester,' I found myself settling into a more peaceful, sustainable existence.

But beneath this otherwise ordinary, if not sympathetic life, there was another layer to my reality that has come to the surface.

For as long as I can remember, I have experienced extraordinary encounters—disturbing, enigmatic, and recurrent. Strange lights that moved with intent. Figures by my bedside that dissolved before I could fully grasp their form. Moments of missing time that left me disoriented and afraid. These experiences shaped my perceptions, infiltrated my dreams, and left me questioning not only their purpose but my own. For years, I carried these fragments without context, unsure whether they were dreams, memories, or something far more unsettling. I lived without the language to explain them—without even the certainty that they had truly happened. But they had. And they were only the beginning.

I've come to think of my life in two separate phases: the world before the encounters, and the world after. Of course, that's an illusion—because the encounters were likely always happening. But my awareness of them came later. And in that early chapter of my life, before anything surfaced, I was like anyone else. I played, I watched cartoons, I chased lightning bugs in the backyard. There was no sense that something strange awaited me. No obvious clue that my life would deviate from the norm.

And yet... I've also come to recognize that even in those "normal" years, there were moments. Subtle ones. Feelings I couldn't name at the time. A particular discomfort with the dark—not the usual fear of monsters under the bed, but something colder. Something less theatrical. I remember feeling, on certain nights, like I was being observed. Not from the hallway or from a closet—but from somewhere else. A vague awareness that the world was thinner than it appeared. That something might be able to step through.

I was a thoughtful kid. Imaginative, but not prone to fantasy. I loved stories, but I was equally fascinated by technology—especially anything futuristic or advanced. I wasn't particularly mechanically inclined, but I was captivated by how things functioned, how systems connected, and how invisible forces—like electricity, gravity, or even time—seemed to govern the world. There's a part of me that wonders whether that curiosity was always in me—or whether it was cultivated. Whether they noticed it early. Whether I was tagged before I even understood what life was.

In school, I was the quiet observer. I made friends easily, but I was never the loud one. I noticed things. When someone was sad. When something didn't make sense. I didn't have words for it back then, but I felt attuned to patterns—especially when they were off. That ability would later become essential in piecing together my own fractured memories.

Looking back now, there's a kind of irony in how long it took me to connect the dots. So much of my early life was structured around helping others feel comfortable—being agreeable, being reliable, being the good son, the good friend, the dependable one. I didn't realize until much later how much of that came from a subconscious desire to anchor myself. To maintain a sense of control. Because somewhere, beneath the surface, I was already being visited. I just hadn't remembered it yet.

That's the strange thing about suppressed memory—it doesn't vanish. It lingers in emotional residue. In unexplained fears. In strange fascinations. I remember watching *Close Encounters of the Third Kind* as a boy, and feeling a chill—not fear exactly, but something deeper. Recognition. I didn't know why that movie affected me the way it did. I do now.

And still, my upbringing was stable. Safe. My parents weren't abusive. There was no trauma I could use to explain the things I'd later recall. In that way, I'm grateful. Because when the memories began to return—when the lights came back, and the beings returned—I couldn't write them off as fantasy born from dysfunction. They didn't come from trauma. They came through it.

So now I'll attempt to frame these experiences against the backdrop of my life—to explore their meaning, their implications, and their origins. A meaning that I hope will not only settle my anxieties but also reveal why these interlopers have been meddling with me and my family for generations.

Origins

I was born in the late 1960s and raised in Des Plaines, Illinois, as the third and youngest son of Norman and Betty Nanstiel. Growing up in the 1970s and '80s, my brothers and I enjoyed a comfortable, middle-class childhood in a friendly subdivision where neighbors knew each other, and children played together without a care. In many ways, my upbringing was a quintessential midwestern suburban existence—free from undue drama, eccentricities, or anything that would suggest my life would be marked by the extraordinary.

Beyond our immediate family in the Chicago area, we were part of a large extended family on both sides—grandparents, aunts, uncles, and cousins—many of whom remained in the suburbs of Pittsburgh, where my parents were born and raised.

I mention them because my story does not begin with me or my garage incident. It begins in 1953 with my mother, Betty, and her family, the Jacksons —with a UFO sighting that may have been the first clue of an extraterrestrial presence woven into our family's history.

1953: Betty and the Incident on Clugston Avenue

My mother, Betty Ann, was nine years old in 1953. She and her seven siblings grew up in the lower-middle-class town of Turtle Creek, Pennsylvania. The family had just moved from the town of Linhart into their Turtle Creek home on Clugston Avenue, a narrow street perched atop Rose Hill, with houses lining one side and a view of a sprawling train yard far below in the valley. Her father, Sidney, had recently purchased the house, which had once been his childhood home.

One night during the summer of that year, after dark, Betty was sitting in the kitchen with her mother, Gertrude, and younger brother Billy when two of her older brothers, Dick and Don, burst in from outside — excited, breathless, and exclaiming that they had seen something remarkable in the sky over the valley.

"Maw! Betty Ann! Don and I just saw a flying saucer above us over the valley!" Dick, the eldest, shouted.

"Calm down. Now say that again?" their mother Gertrude asked, confused but attentive.

"Over the valley!" Dick repeated, Don nodding beside him. *"It*

had colored lights and it was spinning! It hovered for a while above us, out over the train yard, then it shot really fast, straight up and out of sight!"

"Is it gone?" Gertrude asked.

"Yes," Don confirmed. *"It flew up really high and disappeared!"*

Betty and her little brother Billy, eager to verify the sighting, ran through the living room and out the front door onto the covered porch. From there, they could see the open sky above the valley. Dick and Don followed close behind, still buzzing with excitement.

"Where is it?" Betty asked, stepping to the edge of the porch and gazing upward. *"Was it up there?"*

"No, Betty Ann," Dick said. "It was further out — above the train yard."

Betty scanned the sky, disappointed. The stars twinkled overhead, calm and indifferent. Whatever her brothers had seen was gone. Billy, only four years old, looked up beside her with furrowed brows, equally let down. The moment had passed. One by one, they all returned inside to get ready for bed.

The house on Clugston Avenue was a modest, two-story home with three small bedrooms and a creaky wooden staircase. On the ground floor, Sidney and Gertrude slept in a bedroom near the foot of the stairs. Four of Betty's brothers shared the front room upstairs, and Betty slept alone in a smaller room at the back of the house. That night, the windows were open to let in the summer air. The soft hum of insects outside drifted in like a lullaby. The house, once filled with motion and conversation, settled into silence.

Sometime around 2:30 a.m., Betty stirred. She awoke abruptly, not to a sound but to a feeling — a jolt of anxious purpose, as though she'd remembered something urgent. There was no noise in the house. Just the faint creak of the window frame and the occasional rustle of the curtains in the breeze. But inside her, something pressed. She felt pulled.

She sat up slowly, blinking into the dim light of her bedroom. Her heart was already beating faster than it should have been. She wasn't frightened, exactly — just uneasy, as though she had woken up in the middle of something important. There was a thought in her mind that she had to go downstairs. More than a thought — a certainty. She had to check something. Something in the basement.

Moving quietly, she stepped out of bed, padded down the hall and descended the stairs. The air felt heavier the further she went. The living room and kitchen were cast in a soft, sleepy darkness. She turned on a small lamp at the back of the kitchen and paused at the basement door. The feeling persisted — not like a question, but like an instruction.

She opened the door. In that part of Pennsylvania, the hills were rich with coal, and many homes had access to old mine tunnels that ran beneath them. Betty's father had mentioned that their home once connected to one of these mines through the basement. But by the time they moved in, her father had bricked up the mine entrance. Still, the basement was far from welcoming — it was unfinished, with packed dirt underfoot, a rusting furnace, some crude shelving, and a washer. It always smelled of stone, ash, and something faintly metallic. It was not a place any child would want to visit during the day, let alone alone at night.

The light from the kitchen barely reached the bottom of the stairs. Everything surrounding the base of the stairs was shrouded in progressive blackness. She descended slowly, her small hand on the rail. When she reached the third or fourth step, she hesitated, peering into the darkness.

And then she stopped. Something was moving.

She didn't see it clearly — only a stirring at the bottom of the stairs, just beyond the light. Shapes, low and solid. There were two of them. They shifted in tandem, not like people, but like animals. Her body went rigid. She wanted to turn and flee, but her limbs wouldn't respond. The compulsion that had driven her down was gone — replaced by a deep, primal dread.

From the blackness, two German Shepherds stepped into view. They were growling, their lips curled, their eyes fixed on her. She tried to scream, but no sound came. She couldn't move. She couldn't look away. And then — they lunged. Everything went black. What seemed like seconds later, Betty awoke - and she was back in her bed.

She sat up, heart racing, unsure whether she had screamed or gasped. Her bedroom window was still open. The sounds of the summer night returned to her ears slowly, like background noise fading in after a power outage. Her skin was damp. Her hands trembled.

Was it a dream? A nightmare? It hadn't felt like one. Nightmares don't pull you out of bed and place you somewhere else. They don't leave your heart racing like you escaped something real.

Their family had only one dog in 1953 — a small, docile mutt named Fuzzy. Nothing remotely like the animals she had just seen. And certainly nothing in the basement.

The encounter was never repeated. And it was never discussed. For decades, it lived in her memory without explanation — vivid, strange and unresolved. And yet, something from that night stayed with her.

To this day, my mother has an unshakable fear of German Shepherds. She's never had a physical confrontation with one — not before that night, and not since. But the fear is there. Deep and reflexive. Something buried in her body that her mind still can't explain.

The memory lingered in silence, like a bookmark pressed into the spine of a long-forgotten volume, waiting for someone to return to that page. She never forgot it. Not the stillness. Not the stairs. Not the eyes of the creatures that lunged at her. And for a long time, she didn't speak of it to anyone. Until now.

"Fallaces sunt rerum species." (Appearances are deceptive.) – Seneca

I didn't learn of this story from my mother until I began telling her about my own encounters. As I described how my memories were often distorted—how unsettling experiences were disguised in familiar ways—she suddenly recalled the Clugston Avenue incident, a memory she had buried for decades. It had been collecting dust in the attic of her mind, sealed off and unexplained, until something in my words cracked it open.

At first, I called this phenomenon "masked memories," because that's how it felt. As if something alien had put on a human face, slipped into a role I was meant to recognize, and used it as camouflage to move through my awareness undetected. I later discovered that Sigmund Freud had coined a similar concept—screen memories (*Deckerinnerungen*, in German). According to Freud, the human mind itself fabricates these substitute memories as a defense mechanism, shielding the individual from psychic trauma. But in the context of abduction, I don't believe that explanation tells the full story.

I think these screen memories are not internally generated but externally imposed—planted through telepathic suggestion at the moment of trauma, or just before. They're not created by the subconscious to protect us. They're engineered by them, to conceal. To control. A more accurate term, in this context, might be a post-hypnotic veil. That's what it felt like. A haze wrapped around the truth, threaded into my thoughts by something that knew how my mind worked—and how to turn it against itself.

I explained this to my mother and gave her examples from my own experiences. I told her about the times I'd interacted with people I thought were friends or professionals—doctors, airline personnel, even strangers whose presence seemed oddly contextual—only to realize later that I hadn't seen a person at all. My conscious mind had accepted the illusion, as if under a spell. But afterward, as the trance broke, the faces fell apart. The human skin dissolved in memory. What remained behind the mask was something else entirely. What I really saw.

It reminded me of how people make reckless decisions while intoxicated—completely convinced at the time that they're acting rationally—only to see the disaster clearly when the fog lifts. That's what it felt like coming out of these encounters: sobering up from someone else's influence. Only instead of alcohol or drugs, the intoxicant was their control over my perception.

The similarity to hypnosis is hard to ignore. The trance-like states induced during abductions felt far deeper than any meditation or daydream I've ever experienced. There's no gentle descent. One moment, you're there—alert, present—and the next, you're somewhere else entirely, wide-eyed but hollowed out. Your body obeys, your emotions flatten, and your mind stops asking questions. You see what they want you to see. You accept what they want you to believe. And afterward, you struggle to reconstruct what parts were yours, and what were given to you.

One of the most widely cited examples of this phenomenon comes from Whitley Strieber's *Communion* (1986). Strieber recalled seeing a barn owl staring at him through his window—a memory that deeply disturbed him but didn't make sense. Under hypnosis, that image began to unravel. The "owl" was not an owl at all, but a grey. The large, lidless eyes. The unblinking stare. The static presence. The image of the owl had been a kind of placeholder—a screen inserted into his memory, like a mask placed over something his conscious mind was not meant to see.

When I described this to my mother, I saw a look of recognition cross her face. It wasn't just intellectual. It was visceral. I suggested that the German Shepherds she saw at the bottom of the stairs may have been something similar. If greys were present that night, they could have projected the image of the dogs—animals she instinctively feared—to explain the fear and paralysis, to justify the blackout. It would have made the experience emotionally coherent, even if it wasn't true. A planted memory can be more effective than a suppressed one. A frightened child remembers the dogs. She doesn't question what happened in the missing time. But beneath that illusion, something festers. A quiet dissonance. The mind may forget the truth, but the body still feels the angst echoing from the shadows it can't name.

I also told her how, in many reports, the greys often compel the abductee to relocate themselves—usually through telepathic suggestion. A child might rise from bed and wander into an empty room, a backyard, or a basement. Isolated. Separated from others. It's efficient. There's no need for force when the subject is willing, even eager, to follow an impulse they believe is their own. In Betty's case, she may have walked to the basement under that kind of influence. Afterward, I suspect she was guided back upstairs in the same way. This would reduce the chances of memory damage—no jarring discontinuity, just a bizarre dream that fades into the rhythm of an otherwise ordinary childhood.

But that incident isn't the only reason I believe my mother was taken before me. It was just the beginning. Something else happened—something that would reveal itself years later.

And when it did, I couldn't deny what it meant.

2

THE ORBS: SENTINELS OF LIGHT

One morning in the spring of 1970, I awoke before my mother came for me. I don't know what possessed me to stand up inside my crib. Light filtered through the window in pale streaks, soft but insistent, signaling the early morning. It had to be no later than 6:30 a.m.—perhaps even earlier.

The room around me felt still, untouched by the day's motions. I grasped the safety rail, tiny fingers curling around the familiar wooden bars as I pulled myself upright. The mattress beneath my feet sagged slightly with my shifting weight, but the crinkling of the plastic soles on my one-piece pajamas gave me something to anchor myself to—a tangible, reassuring texture in a world that was still so new. I took in my surroundings, my baby-blue walls a gentle contrast to the glow of morning. A mobile—one of my first possessions—dangled motionlessly above the diaper-changing table.

I don't remember what I had been thinking in those moments, standing there alone in my crib, but I remember looking toward the closet door.

And I remember the Orb.

A white, glowing mass of plasma - about the size of a softball - slid effortlessly through the door, its form defying the solid boundary as though the wooden structure meant nothing. It didn't make a sound—no creak of the hinges, no rush of air. Just motion, smooth and deliberate.

I was sixteen months old. I didn't know what fear was. I didn't even have the capacity to question what I was seeing. The whole world was new to me, filled with strange, incomprehensible things. And so I simply watched it.

My eyes fixated on this luminous intruder as it crossed the room toward me, its glow reflecting off the baby-blue walls, casting subtle shadows in places that should have had none. It moved no faster than a slow adult's walk, unhurried, as if it had all the time in the world.

And then, it was with me. The Orb reached my forehead and I was rendered unconscious.

The Recurring Visits

That was the first encounter I remember. And from that morning in 1970 until sometime in 1974, it happened again, many times.

I don't know why I remembered these visits when so many other early memories from childhood faded into nothingness. But this remained. It became a pattern, a part of my reality for four years that had no explanation.

When my bedroom was still in what would later become my parents' dining room, the Orb would always emerge from the closet. Later, when my bed was moved upstairs to the second floor, I would watch it come through the knee-wall adjacent to the ceiling, defying every law of matter I would later be taught in school. And always, it moved the same way—steady, controlled, intentional. It never hesitated, faltered or wavered. I was its target.

Each time, I would feel that familiar rush of awareness, staring wide-eyed at the glowing anomaly. And each time, it would reach my forehead— I would black out as though my brain were controlled by a switch.

But while I would always lose consciousness, I never lost the memories. And over time, those memories took on a different shape.

As the years passed, I began to fear closets—in any room, in any house. The fear wasn't rational, not the way a child fears the dark or the imagined monsters beneath the bed. It was deeply ingrained, embedded in my subconscious in a way that existed without explanation. An enduring angst, emerging from the shadows. It lived in the periphery of my awareness - a feeling that something waited just beyond the edges of ordinary life.

I didn't know why I was afraid or what it meant. But I knew the feeling. The suddenness. The aggression. The way the Orb would enter my space with purpose, and unwavering determination. I knew that whatever it was, it was not a dream. And that it would return.

1974

The age of five was the final year when I remember receiving visits from the white plasma orb. The most notable of these visits occurred when I was toward the end of a four-night hospital stay at Lutheran General in Park Ridge, IL. A few months prior, I had sustained a concussion in an inflatable bounce house, where I had fallen and was trampled by a few other children. For a few years, post injury, I had some difficulties with petit mal seizures, which I outgrew before puberty. For reasons related, I was undergoing tests at the hospital and was admitted for observation for the duration of these tests.

On my last night at Lutheran General, I remember laying down for sleep in the bed closest to the door and bathroom, with my roommate Tommy in the bed adjacent to the windows with a view of Dempster street, several stories below our room. Tommy was critically sick with an infected abscess in his abdomen, and had a high fever between 105 and 110. He was connected to IV's and placed on an ice mattress to cool him down and often had his mother by his side, even as he slept. It was unknown if he would survive the night. He was usually unconscious and too sick to hold conversation, so I left him in peace.

Before I could fall asleep, in the darkened room, I was staring at the door to the hallway. The top half of the door had a wire-reinforced glass window, covered by white linen curtains. While the room was mostly dark, light was visible from the hallway if you looked in that direction. I was calm as my breathing lengthened and was relaxed enough to begin drifting to sleep.

Just then, as I was still looking at the room's only source of light, the white orb reappeared by moving through the door, from the hallway, and toward my bed. As with previous encounters, it moved at the speed of a person walking, until it reached my forehead and I once again passed unconscious. I awoke next morning with the sun's rays exploiting the gaps at the edges of the closed curtains, filling the room with subdued light, where I could observe Tommy, still asleep with his mother at his side.

After the nurse had come in to check on Tommy and me, I had used the restroom and was awaiting my mother who was coming to take me home that morning. I was excited to leave. I was there for four days and hated the hospital for the uncomfortable environment it was.

When my mother arrived to gather me for the trip home, I remember her standing in the doorway of our room with the light of the hallway spilling in. The outer window curtains were still drawn, so the hallway was relatively bright compared to our room. Her purse was slung over her right shoulder, and she was holding an object in her right hand. She asked me to gather my things so we could leave. All I had with me to gather was my plush toy bunny rabbit I had named "hopper," and some match box cars I had received as a gift to amuse me during my hospital stay. Once I had collected my belongings and joined my mother, Tommy's mom walked over to us to say farewell, and exchanged phone numbers as they had spoken a few times since the day before.

Once they had exchanged numbers, I learned what my mother was holding in her right hand. It was a toy truck she had purchased for Tommy at the hospital's gift shop. "Here, Erik, go say goodbye to Tommy and give him this present." my mother told me. As I had felt uncomfortable around Tommy for the duration of my stay, I objected. "I don't want to talk to him, Mommy. He's going to die!" While nobody told me he was deathly ill, I felt it instinctually. But my mother objected to my disdain. "Erik, you have to say goodbye to him! It's the nice thing to do!"

Rolling my eyes in mild exasperation, I relented. "Okay, fine!" I accepted the truck from my mother's hand and walked over to Tommy's bed. Next to his bed was a small wooden three-stepped set of stairs that was placed for Tommy to climb in and out of bed. I used the stairs to climb to the top step and observed Tommy looking at me. I placed his toy truck on the bed beside him, said nothing and spread both my hands with my fingers as wide apart as I could make them, laying my hands on Tommy's abdomen, then slowly moved them up and down his torso. Tommy didn't flinch, as he was weak and exhausted. I was aware of my mother and Tommy's mom watching me in confused curiosity, and as a result I felt a little self conscious as I proceeded.

In that moment, I was acting out of pure instinct. Somehow, I knew with zero doubt that I could heal this boy with my hands. But I was only doing it because my mother said I had to be nice to him. I still didn't want to talk to him, but when I had finished I had dismissed myself by exclaiming "There! Now you're going to be all better!"

That moment, I climbed down from Tommy's side and rejoined my mother as we exited the room. I could hear my mother and Tommy's mom promise to keep in touch as I ran ahead down the hallway, looking admiringly at my hands. "I have magic hands!" I exclaimed. Why did I think this? Nobody suggested to me that someone other than Jesus could do such a thing. But that's where my mind was at.

Years later, this incident came up as my mother told me the story of how the next day, Tommy's mother called her with an amazing revelation. After we said our goodbyes, Tommy was examined by his doctors who found that Tommy's fever had disappeared. After some tests, they verified that the large, infected abscess inside his abdomen that was killing him, was completely gone. His vital signs were now perfectly normal. And no sign of infection remained. Tommy's mother called it a miracle and credited my actions as she spoke to my mom. I have always wondered what happened to Tommy in the years since. I never learned his surname.

Though I didn't understand it at the time, and didn't make the connection until decades later, I now believe the white orb's visit to my hospital room may have been about more than just monitoring. It's possible that what I witnessed that night—and what followed the next day—was not just a passive visitation, but a deliberate act of healing. Not just of observation, but intervention.

I wasn't aware of other cases like mine until much later, after I began researching the phenomenon in earnest. What I found startled me. There exists a body of reports from other abductees and experiencers who, like me, described unexplained healing following encounters with glowing orbs. These orbs—usually described as white, bluish, or sometimes golden—have been seen entering hospital rooms, hovering over the bodies of the sick, and even interacting with unconscious or dying patients. In many of these accounts, witnesses reported profound and often medically inexplicable recoveries afterward.

In *The Healing Power of UFOs*, researcher Preston Dennett documents over a hundred such cases. In one striking account, a man suffering from terminal cancer awoke in the middle of the night to find a glowing orb floating above his bed. It hovered silently for a few moments, then moved slowly over his chest and abdomen before vanishing. The next day, his pain had subsided. Within weeks, his scans showed no sign of cancer. The case baffled his doctors. There was no scientific explanation for his recovery.

In another account cited by Dennett, a young woman recovering from spinal surgery reported a glowing ball of light entering her hospital room late at night. She described it as having an intelligent presence, something that felt "aware." The orb hovered over her surgical incision for several minutes, during which she experienced a tingling sensation throughout her body. By morning, her pain was gone. The incision had healed at an accelerated rate. Again, the doctors were stunned.

The similarity to my experience is unsettling. I had received a concussion months prior and was in the hospital for seizure monitoring and post-injury testing. While I don't remember the orb making physical contact, I do recall that it approached my forehead directly—just before I blacked out. This precise motion had occurred in all previous encounters. It was never random. It moved toward me with purpose. At the time, I interpreted it with the innocent curiosity of a child, but now I see it differently. Perhaps that moment was not only about observation. Perhaps it triggered something in me—or through me.

I think often of what I did the next morning, when I instinctively laid my hands on Tommy and declared, "Now you're going to be all better." I had no reference point for that kind of behavior. I wasn't raised to believe in mystical healing, and nobody had ever modeled that for me. Yet I acted with absolute certainty, as if something had been placed within me—a sense of knowing that wasn't mine to begin with. A child's impulse, yes, but one carried out with the kind of purpose that still echoes in my memory.

Could the orb have activated something within me that allowed Tommy's body to recover? Or had it acted on Tommy directly, and I was simply a witness—or a symbolic conduit—for something already underway? Perhaps the act of healing wasn't performed through my hands, but was instead orchestrated through me, just as I had been watched, tracked, and influenced in ways I did not understand. This kind of influence—the ability to heal through non-human intervention—has been cited by researchers such as Dr. John Mack and Budd Hopkins. Both men interviewed abductees who reported physical or psychological improvements following contact, especially after being exposed to strange light or energy fields.

At the time, I didn't know any of this. I only knew that I had done something extraordinary—and that Tommy's recovery, though joyful, carried a strange and heavy silence. No one could explain it. No one tried.

But now, with the benefit of hindsight, I see that my earliest interactions with the orbs may have involved more than mere surveillance. I may have been a participant in something far more complex—something that defied the limits of conventional medicine and biology. Something that began not with fear, but with healing.

Why, you might ask, am I sharing this story about Tommy and I? Healing someone with one's hands is usually within the realm of religious and spiritual faith. But I feel it's necessary to tell this story, given that it happened within hours of a visit from the white plasma orb. I am taking this experience within the context of my encounters. And when you read about one of my later encounters as an adult, whereby I had experienced a healing at the hands of my abductors, you'll better understand my need to associate them with Tommy's healing.

For much of my life, I never made a connection between these glowing orbs and anything beyond the immediate experiences themselves. To me, they were simply a recurring anomaly—something unexplained but not necessarily linked to a larger phenomenon. It wasn't until 2020—when my encounters with the Greys became undeniable—that I began investigating the abduction phenomenon in earnest. That was when I discovered something startling: these white plasma orbs have been widely reported by others who claim similar encounters.

Many abductees have described orbs of light appearing before, during, or after their experiences. These orbs—often seen as bright white, bluish, or occasionally orange—move in deliberate, controlled ways, sometimes even passing through walls, ceilings, or people themselves. Some witnesses report losing time or experiencing paralysis immediately after an orb appears, while others describe feeling an eerie sense of being observed.

Historical Reports of Plasma Orbs in UFO and Abduction Phenomena

The British Ministry of Defence's "Project Condign" (1997–2000) explored the idea that some UFO sightings and orb encounters may be caused by highly charged plasma formations. Their findings suggested that these energy fields might induce altered states of consciousness in witnesses, potentially explaining missing time or memory gaps.

But some researchers argue that plasma orbs are more than just natural energy anomalies. Harvard psychiatrist Dr. John Mack, who studied hundreds of abductees, documented numerous cases in which witnesses recalled seeing floating orbs either before, during, or after their encounters. Some described them as intelligent, with a presence that felt "watchful."

In the famous Skinwalker Ranch case in Utah, glowing orbs have been repeatedly reported by military personnel and researchers alike. Some claim the orbs followed them, reacted to their movements, or even induced physiological effects. Similarly, in Hessdalen, Norway, and the Marfa Lights in Texas, persistent reports describe luminous orbs behaving in ways that seem more deliberate than random natural phenomena.

Were the Orbs in My Childhood More Than Just Energy?

If these orbs were more than just random anomalies, then what was their purpose? Could they have been marking me in some way, preparing me for something yet to come? And if they appeared so frequently in my early life, were they also present for my mother?

It's possible, however, that these orbs were not merely separate entities or remote observation devices—but Greys themselves, cloaked in a different form.

Many abductees, including myself, have witnessed Greys moving through solid objects like walls and ceilings, an ability that suggests they have the technology to alter their density, molecular structure, or dimensional state. If that's the case, then what if the plasma orbs aren't separate objects at all, but rather the Greys themselves in a cloaked phase? Using some electrogravitic technology that can render them effectively massless?

This would explain why they move with intelligence rather than behaving like natural energy phenomena, why they approach individuals directly, and why contact with them results in immediate unconsciousness, as if transitioning into another state of interaction. Their tendency to precede abductions suggests they are not passive observers but rather an integral part of the process. If Greys can phase through matter, then perhaps when they do, they appear as these plasma orbs. Their luminescence might not be a coincidence but rather a visible effect of their cloaking technology.

At this point, I don't have definitive answers. But the presence of these glowing orbs in my early life suggests that my involvement in this phenomenon began long before I was old enough to recognize it.

A Second Sign of Generational Contact

1974 was not only the final year I witnessed the glowing orbs that visited me—it was also the year my mother, Betty, began experiencing a series of vivid, disturbing, and recurrent dreams that, in retrospect, seem impossible to dismiss as mere imagination.

In these dreams, my mother, my father, and I were visiting friends just four houses away from our own. As we stepped outside to walk home, hundreds of bright white orbs descended from the sky. They weren't just appearing—they were pursuing us. My father and mother decided we should run, taking cover by sneaking from backyard to backyard, trying desperately to make it home. But no matter how carefully we moved, the orbs were relentless. Each time we emerged from behind a tree, a shed, or a fence, they had closed the distance. They were hunting us.

Before we could reach our house, the orbs finally overtook us, surrounding us in a blinding white light. My mother froze in fear as a brilliant spotlight enveloped her. In this moment, my father turned to her and said, "Don't worry, honey, they just want to make you into an angel." And then—I was gone.

Each time she had this dream, it ended the same way: I had vanished. Betty would awaken in a panic, shaken by the dream's eerie consistency. To this day—51 years later—she still remembers these dreams with unsettling clarity.

A Subconscious Cry for the Truth?

I include my mother's dreams in this memoir because, given the context of my own encounters, they seem like more than just an overactive imagination. It is difficult to ignore the implications: she had these dreams during the exact same period that I was witnessing the white orbs in my room. Not only that, but the dream itself mirrors the same kind of pursuit and eventual capture that I later experienced in my own abductions.

Had my mother also been experiencing her own visitations—without a waking memory of them? Was she subconsciously aware that I was being taken, even if she had no conscious recollection of it?

It is also important to consider the cultural context of the time. These dreams predate any major Hollywood influence on the abduction phenomenon. *Close Encounters of the Third Kind* wouldn't be released for another three years. *E.T. the Extra-Terrestrial* was still eight years away. The last significant wave of UFO-related pop culture had been in the 1950s—twenty years prior.

Beyond that, my mother has never been interested in science fiction. She actively dislikes the genre. There was nothing in popular culture that could have planted such imagery in her mind.

Given all this, I cannot help but believe that my mother's involvement was not limited to what happened in 1953. She may have been visited long after the Clugston Avenue incident, and possibly even alongside me, without consciously realizing it.

If that's the case, then how much did she truly know, even if only on a subconscious level?

A mother's intuition is powerful—an almost primal instinct when it comes to protecting a child. If she was being visited alongside me, it's possible that, while awake, she remained unaware of what was happening. But something deep inside her must have recognized the pattern, must have sensed that I was being taken. These dreams—occurring over and over again—suggest an awareness that she could not articulate consciously, but one her mind refused to release.

She never recalled seeing the white orbs in waking life. Yet there they were, pursuing her in her dreams—a relentless force she could never outrun. How does a person dream of something they've never seen? If the orbs were imprinted in her subconscious, does that mean she had once witnessed them, only to have the memory buried?

The most haunting part of her dream is its conclusion. Every single time, I disappeared.

Her fear wasn't for herself; it was for me. Even in this altered dream world, where the boundaries between memory and imagination blurred, her mind consistently played out the same outcome: the orbs took me, and she was left behind to wake in panic. What does that say about what she truly understood?

Most abductees struggle with isolation—the maddening impossibility of proving what has happened to them. But what if the proof has always been there, not as clear memories, but as imprints left in the minds of those closest to us? How many other abductees have family members who have sensed their disappearances in ways they don't consciously understand? How many parents, spouses, or siblings have been haunted by unexplained dreams, flashes of fear, or moments of inexplicable grief—without ever realizing what they were mourning?

These visitations don't just affect individuals. They ripple outward, embedding themselves in families, spanning generations, subtly altering the course of our lives without us even realizing it. If my mother was dreaming of these events while I was experiencing them, then my abductions weren't just my reality. They were hers, too.

She may not have been able to remember. But she knew. And that, more than anything, tells me that what happened to me was never going to be kept a secret forever.

Looking back, I realize how strange it is that my earliest experiences with the unknown were not rooted in terror or pain, but in something far more ambiguous—something that held both beauty and violation in equal measure. The orbs were not violent. They did not scream, chase, or harm in any conventional sense. And yet, their presence altered me. They entered my space without permission.

They crossed thresholds meant to keep me safe. They rendered me unconscious and reappeared again and again with a purpose I could never see, only feel. They marked me. And in doing so, they rewrote the foundation of what I believed reality could be.

For many years, I believed those visits ended in 1974. I told myself that the orb simply stopped coming after that final hospital encounter. But the truth, as I would come to understand decades later, is that the nature of the visits changed. They evolved. What began with light would later take form. What began as a glowing presence would later reveal itself as beings who no longer needed to hide behind radiance. They stepped out of the light—and into the room.

I don't know why I was chosen. I don't know if Tommy was meant to be healed, or if I was meant to believe that I had done the healing. Perhaps both. But what I do know is that I wasn't just a witness to these events. I was a participant. However small, however young, I was involved in something beyond explanation. Something that would follow me for the rest of my life.

And my mother—whether by intuition or by her own suppressed experiences—was entangled in it too. Her dreams were not warnings. They were echoes. Refractions of what was really happening behind the veil of normal life. And the orbs were the first breach of that veil.

I now see those orbs not as anomalies, but as sentinels—scouts of a larger intelligence that would later reveal itself more clearly. They weren't random. They were preparatory. And while I didn't know it then, those early encounters laid the groundwork for everything that would come next. What began in light would one day return in form.

3
THROUGH A GLASS, DARKLY

In the twenty years following, nothing related to UFO's or abduction encounters had happened to me, of which I'm aware. I spent 1975 until 1987 going through the grades of public schooling, living my very normal midwestern, suburban life. I was enjoying my family and my friends as I made mostly-pleasant, life-long memories. From 1987 until the early 1990's, I attended college at Iowa State University and studied English as a major, with an emphasis on technical writing and communication. I also took several electives in the sciences, including astronomy and physics as I had always held a fascination for what lies beyond our world, in the universe. To this day, I'm often watching documentaries about galaxies, exoplanets, black holes and all manner of stellar phenomena. The mysteries of the world are not confined to our terrestrial existence. And my wonder has always reached out into the stellar void as I attempted to understand what it is to be us and where we may be headed in a future I may never see. My brothers never had such compulsions. Nor have my childhood friends. Why have I? Why did I thirst for the esoteric unknown?

By 1994, I had moved from my parents' home to an apartment in Wheeling, Illinois with my best friend, Joe Witkowski. We shared a two bedroom apartment. I was working at a trade magazine publisher in Des Plaines as a graphic production employee, while Joe was working as a traveling forklift technician. It was fun to finally be independent of my parents and stretch my wings as a young adult. As I settled into my life and the freedom of adulthood, I was about to experience something new. Something I couldn't understand until recently.

For nearly twenty years, the mysteries of my childhood had faded into the background. I had no memories of abductions, no strange orbs appearing in my room, nothing to suggest that the unknown had any further claim on me. I had grown up, gone to college, and built a life with the belief that whatever happened in my early years—if anything truly happened at all—was firmly in the past. I had moved forward, completely unaware that I was merely in an intermission rather than an ending.

The past wasn't finished with me. On an ordinary Saturday morning in August 1994, something happened that I couldn't ignore.

1994

On August 20th, the third Saturday of the month, I was asleep in bed around 6:30 a.m. when I found myself entering a lucid stage of REM sleep. Lucid dreaming is a strange threshold—where one is asleep but aware of the fact and can sometimes influence the dream's direction. At that moment, I recognized the opportunity. I could either stay immersed and conjure something whimsical to explore, or I could simply awaken and begin my day. I chose the latter. I had plans, and I wanted an early start.

But despite this intention, something unexpected seized control of my awareness. A new dream began to unfold, not born of my imagination, but forced upon me. It felt like an imposed visual overlay—like a hijacked channel broadcast into my mind. Above my field of view, I saw a maple leaf suspended in the sunlight. It was green and pristine, its delicate veins and cellular structure illuminated in radiant detail as the sun poured through it. And oddly, I seemed to rotate beneath the leaf, as if I were weightless, tumbling slowly in place. A haunting, wind-up melody accompanied the scene—like the tune of an old music box, sweet and artificial, looping with an unsettling consistency. It might have been beautiful if it hadn't felt so wrong.

Even in that state, I could tell something was off. I had intended to wake myself, but this vision had elbowed its way into my consciousness, like a distraction designed to hold me in place. It wasn't mine. That recognition alone shifted my awareness. Though my eyes remained closed, I began to register sounds from the physical world. The steady hum of my floor fan was there, offering its usual white noise, but layered beneath it, I heard movement—rustling fabric on both sides of the bed. Soft brushing sounds, like clothing sliding across bedding. Someone—maybe more than one—was in my room.

A jolt of panic surged through me. I tried to open my eyes but couldn't. My body wouldn't respond. I was paralyzed, locked in place by some unseen force. The imagery of the leaf continued, vivid and unwelcome, as if trying to pacify me with serenity while my instincts screamed otherwise. I fought back, forcing my will against whatever was holding me down. My muscles tensed. I began to thrash slightly under the strain. The mattress trembled beneath me as I struggled. And then—suddenly—it broke. I snapped free.

My eyes burst open, and I bolted upright, gasping. My head jerked to the left just in time to catch a sight I'll never forget: four small, humanoid figures, slender and uniformed in black coveralls, whooshing out of my room like shadows fleeing a spotlight. They moved in perfect synchronization—one after the other—propelled with impossible speed. Whoosh, whoosh, whoosh, whoosh. They didn't run. They didn't walk. They glided—or were yanked—like marionettes pulled by invisible strings.

Even in that fraction of a second, I could make out features. Large, pale heads with bulbous craniums. Smooth, ashen-grey skin. Enormous black eyes that seemed to drink in all available light. White, delicate hands emerged from the sleeves of their suits. They had a humanoid form, but they weren't human. Their appearance was clinical, precise. Inhumanly deliberate.

The door to my room had been closed. But that didn't matter. One by one, they passed through it as if it wasn't there—phasing through solid matter without resistance, like spirits or holograms made real. There was no dramatic flash, no sound of impact. Just their abrupt disappearance into whatever lay beyond that door.

I sat there stunned, my nerves vibrating with electricity. My jaw hung open, my heart pounding so hard I could hear it in my ears. I didn't chase them—not because I didn't want to, but because my body was frozen in the kind of astonished stillness that only raw disbelief can cause. My first and only thought was "What just happened?" Had I dreamed it? Was it real? How could anything move that fast?

I couldn't confide in Joe, my roommate and best friend, because he wasn't home that weekend. His job as a mobile forklift technician often had him flying across the country, tools in tow, servicing equipment in warehouses and factories. His room, just steps away, was empty. I longed to knock on his door, just to ask, "Did you see that?" Not because I expected validation, but because I desperately needed it.

Later that day, I called my father and shared the story. I needed to say it out loud, to get it out of my system. As I recall, he simply said, "Whoa." He didn't dismiss it, but he didn't probe either. What else could he say? We didn't linger on the subject. The conversation moved on, and the weight of the moment receded. I had nothing to add—no context, no memory of previous experiences to tie it to. So I let it fade.

But that wasn't the last strange thing to happen that year.

Not long afterward—weeks, maybe a couple months—I had another experience, though at the time I interpreted it very differently. It didn't feel like an abduction. It felt like a lucid dream. But now, I'm not so sure.

One morning, I found myself in a lucid state of consciousness, somewhere between dreaming and waking. Everything was black at first, until I became aware that someone was leaning over me. A face appeared—upside down in my field of view, hovering over mine, her hands positioned just beside each of my ears. I couldn't feel her touch, but I felt the heat of her palms, as if she was radiating energy. I recognized her instantly. It was Leslie Krowka, a beloved family friend and neighbor of my parents. She had passed away years earlier, and seeing her again filled me with surprise and emotion.

"Leslie!" I said. "What are you doing here? You've been gone so long. Everybody loves you and misses you." She didn't smile. She just looked at me with calm, unwavering eyes and said something that stayed with me for decades.

"Mary misses you."

"Mary?" I asked. "Who is Mary? I don't know anyone named Mary."

"It is she who sent me to you," Leslie replied.

That phrasing struck me immediately. *It is she...* Who talks like that? It felt formal, ritualistic—like a messenger delivering a decree. The moment was brief. I woke up suddenly, fully alert, sitting up in bed. I knew it hadn't been an ordinary dream. It had a presence. A weight. I felt that I'd been visited.

At the time, I thought it was a spiritual event—a message from the other side. But in retrospect, I can't say that with certainty. In fact, the more I think about it, the less sense it makes. If Mary was someone in the spiritual realm who missed me, why didn't she come herself? Why send Leslie? Why such stiff, impersonal language?

I never told anyone about that moment—not until now. I truly believed it was a spiritual encounter. But the years have complicated that interpretation. I can't help but wonder if it was something else entirely—something more calculated.

Why would a familiar face appear in a dream that felt more sent than imagined? Why would the message come from someone I hadn't seen in years, using formal language that felt scripted rather than heartfelt? And who was Mary?

I don't have the answers. But looking back through the lens of all I've experienced since, I can't ignore the possibility that this moment may have been another layer of the same phenomenon—masked, softened, and delivered in a form meant to bypass resistance. Whether it was spiritual or constructed, I only know this: it was not mine. And it has never left me.

If either of these events had occurred in isolation—never to repeat—I might've chalked them up to anomalies of the mind. The first could be explained away as a vivid case of sleep paralysis—a hypnopompic hallucination, which affects an estimated 12% of the population. These episodes often involve the terrifying sensation of waking while paralyzed, accompanied by realistic auditory or visual phenomena. What I experienced that morning could easily be filed in that category. In fact, for years, that's exactly what I did.

The second—what I took to be a spiritual visitation—felt entirely different, yet no less strange. At the time, I didn't place it within the same framework. I made no connection between Leslie's appearance and what I'd seen earlier that year. And I certainly didn't associate it with the orbs of light from my childhood, which I had long since filed away as something symbolic or surreal. Those were dreamlike fragments from an age when reality was still malleable. In contrast, these new experiences felt tangible. Unsettling. Concrete. But since nothing else happened—at least, not in any way I could consciously recall—I moved on.

And yet, something in me never truly forgot. Something remained open, unresolved, waiting for the day when it would all begin to make sense.

1995

A year later, my best friend Joseph and I had decided to part as roommates, as he had met a woman he was serious about and wanted to take their next steps together. I found a new apartment in the same town of Wheeling, Illinois - a single bedroom that I had moved into by mid January. It wasn't as fun to be living on my own, but the apartment was affordable and I was happy that I had enough furniture and appliances to fill it.

This was a year that I considered particularly lonesome. On weekends, I would often drive out to my brother's house that he and his wife owned in Lake in the Hills, IL - where we would party a few weekends a month. I enjoyed drinking and laughing with my brother Ron and his wife Milly. And they had a comfortable couch I could crash on if I became inebriated. I was 26 years old and was still in the youth-mindset that socializing and partying on weekends was the thing to do. But even that, as a distraction, became old hat after a time. I'd say most of the weekends that I visited them for socializing was in the first third of the year. By that summer, I had begun spending more time alone in my apartment where I found myself doing a lot of reading and writing down various ideas I had.

During this year, I cannot recall any overt abduction encounters. Nothing like the experience I had a year earlier where I startled the four greys by waking suddenly - and witnessed them leaving my room in a hurry. As I had mentioned I was doing a lot of reading, and I had taken interest in a book that my father had given me - that was once in his father's library, a 1929 book entitled *"The Projection of the Astral Body"* by Sylvan Muldoon and Hereward Carrington. The copy I had was a revised edition published in 1947. I was interested in it because I wanted to attempt to project myself "astrally" - where one can train themselves to separate their soul from their body... while conscious. What can I say? I had a lot of time on my hands.

As I pursued this effort, one of the techniques outlined in the book was to train oneself to awaken every night at the same time... I chose 2:45 a.m. This was normally a time where I would be deeply asleep. Each morning at that precise time, my alarm would sound and I would wake up, douse the alarm and practice a meditation. These meditations would involve giving myself a post-hypnotic suggestion... with the premise that waking during the deepest parts of sleep would already afford me the deepest of relaxations and proper brain activity for an entranced state. The suggestion I would give myself was that I would separate from my body and float above it while conscious. And I did this for several weeks. Eventually, my brain began entering a partial waking state before the alarm went off.

And having rehearsed the same mantra of "I'm going to separate from my body tonight" or some such phrase, the idea became a subconscious directive.

Then, one night, I became conscious with my eyes closed and I could feel myself tearing away from my body which was lying on its right side. The separation felt similar to the sensation of tearing velcro apart. And the sound was similar also. Would you like an example of how it sounded? If you've ever watched the movie "Ghost" with Patrick Swayze and Demi Moore, there was a sound effect the movie used every time a ghost passed slowly through something or someone. That was the closest analog to the experience itself. And here I was, feeling myself floating outward as I lay on my right side. And it couldn't have been more than a few feet. Because at that point, the sensation made me feel extremely vulnerable - which snapped my mind to full alert, interrupting the experience. I snapped back with a shudder. Breathing heavily and opening my eyes as I darted my head about the room.

On another occasion I woke up already outside my body as I was lying on my back. The textured stucco of the concrete ceiling above me was inches from my eyes! Disembodied, I was floating by the ceiling! And as before, I felt scared and snapped back with a shudder only to awaken fully as the experience ended. I decided that was the last time I would want to experience that. It is difficult to describe how vulnerable that feels. The closest analogy I have is when I'm outside in a large field as a lightning storm approaches overhead. My only thought is to get to the safety of the indoors and not be the tallest thing around me as lightning flashes above me. On July 4, 1994 I once witnessed lightning obliterate a tree just 50 yards from where I stood, in Des Plaines, IL. From that moment on, I couldn't handle being outside during a storm. So, by comparison, you could call my aversion to "astral projection" a kind of phobia.

I mention these experiences because they preceded a unique incident I had that gave me a clue that I may have been visited during this period of time. But I cannot be certain. One night, some time in July of 1995 I became lucid during my sleep. I wasn't dreaming any imagery - everything was dark in my view. My eyes were still closed, but my mind was very conscious. Knowing I was in a kind of hypnotic, waking state, I spontaneously asked a question that had no precedent or forethought. I asked "I wonder if THEY could show me what God looks like?"

Now, looking back, I had no reason to think of a "they" in my life. Who are "they?" Why would I ask any "they" for anything? But my subconscious mind had access to my waking mind. And it wanted to know if "they" - whoever that might be - could show me what God looked like.

As soon as I tried to answer my own question with a "no, THEY wouldn't do that" an image bounded into my mind - stark, startling and very fearsome.

In the brightest, living color of magenta, I witnessed what appeared as a line-drawing of a great eye with outstretched feathered wings. And behind it, a series of concentric rectangles that radiated from the center behind it, outward. And these rectangles seemed to pulsate with energy from the center, outward. So the bright, neon-magenta color would intensify for each of these nested rectangles as the energy wave pulsed to the outer rectangles. I had never seen anything like this before. But more than this imagery, was the intelligence and the sheer power behind it. This image was LIVING, for the lack of a better description. I felt it KNOWING me and there was this powerful bass hum like a low rumble that penetrated into my soul. I felt genuine fear and awe to witness this being - whatever it was. The vision lasted about 15 seconds.

At that time, in 1995, I had never seen anything like that symbol. But I surmised, that as a symbol, the eye represented all knowing omniscience as the wings represented omnipresence and power. So if any culture were to have a symbol for a God that fit human allegories, a winged eye would be perfect, wouldn't it?

Some time later, I ran across a book of Egyptian artwork and saw this symbol! The Egyptians had a winged sun-disk, often associated with Horus or Ra, positioned atop temples and engraved in ancient reliefs. My heart skipped. The resemblance was immediate and undeniable. It was the same fundamental image that had appeared to me in my sleep—an all-seeing presence with feathered wings. But what unsettled me even more was its antiquity.

The Egyptians were not the first to use this symbol. As I dug deeper, I found that the Sumerians had an earlier version of it, one linked to the Anunnaki, the so-called "gods" of Mesopotamian civilization. Their depiction carried the same defining traits—a central disk with outstretched wings, sometimes containing a figure inside, other times an eye-like emblem. It was a symbol of cosmic authority, appearing above kings, temples, and in celestial narratives. In every culture where this imagery appeared, it represented divine rule, omniscience, and control. The Egyptians linked it to the sun, kingship, and the gods' omnipresence over the mortal world. The Mesopotamians associated it with the Anunnaki, celestial overseers who descended from the sky. The Babylonians and Assyrians incorporated it into their depictions of Marduk and Ashur, reinforcing the idea that this was not just a religious symbol—it was a mark of governance, surveillance, and dominance.

But then something struck me—the concentric rectangles I had seen pulsating outward behind the winged eye. At first, I had assumed they were a framing device, a way of emphasizing the image's intensity. But then a new perspective dawned on me. What if these weren't just geometric shapes? The stacked, nested pattern was eerily reminiscent of something else: a pyramid viewed from directly above. If that's the case, then this symbol didn't just represent divinity or power; it was connected to an architectural form that has stood as an enigma for millennia. The idea of a winged sun hovering over a pyramid aligns almost too well with ancient depictions of celestial authority and knowledge descending to earth.

At the time, I didn't have an answer. But the more I researched, the more questions multiplied. The Book of Ezekiel described the ophanim—wheels within wheels, covered in eyes, moving in ways beyond human comprehension. Some believe Ezekiel was witnessing something technological, not supernatural. The seraphim, divine beings of fire with multiple wings, bear an eerie resemblance to the radiating, pulsating nature of the symbol I saw. The Eye of Providence, found in esoteric traditions from Masonic lodges to Rosicrucian orders, is another variation of this archetype—an omnipotent force watching from above. Had humanity's concept of divine oversight been seeded by actual encounters? Had ancient cultures merely interpreted advanced aerial phenomena through the limited framework of their time? And if so, were the Greys part of this equation? Had they shown me something that predated our written history?

There is another possibility—one that unnerves me even more. What if this vision wasn't meant to answer my question? What if it was meant to remind me of something I had forgotten? When I asked if "they" could show me what God looked like, I wasn't consciously thinking of the Greys. At the time, I wasn't even considering myself an abductee. But my subconscious knew exactly who to ask. That alone is worth contemplating. Had I seen this symbol before, somewhere beyond conscious recollection? Was it something shown to me during an encounter I no longer remembered? If the Greys were responsible for placing this vision in my mind, then they not only knew this symbol but found it significant enough to project it into my awareness at a pivotal moment. And if that's the case, why? Was it simply an acknowledgment, a way of reinforcing their role as watchers, as the ones in control? Or was it something more, something tied to a deeper reality that humanity has only ever glimpsed through mythology and religious interpretation?

The implications haunted me. If the Greys are part of this long-standing presence, then their involvement in human history runs far deeper than simple genetic experiments. They are not just visitors. They may be the architects of something far older. The vision left me with more questions than answers. But one thing was certain: even in my quietest moments, something was still watching. And, just as before, I had no way of knowing when they would return.

It wasn't until many years later that the vision returned to me in an unexpected way—triggered not by another encounter, but by something far more mundane. At a local craft fair, I happened to notice a child's yarn project hanging from a vendor's rack—brightly colored thread wrapped in layers around two crossed sticks, forming a pattern of nested concentric squares. I froze. It hit me with eerie familiarity. Though there was no winged eye, the geometry—square upon square radiating from a center point—was unmistakable. It mirrored the vision I had seen in 1995, behind the great magenta eye. But this was labeled Ojo de Dios—Spanish for "God's Eye."

I had never looked into them before, but I learned that these were sacred artifacts in their original context—woven by the Huichol and other Indigenous peoples of Mexico and South America. The central point represented divine sight, while the surrounding squares symbolized layers of perception or expanding spiritual insight. They were created to offer protection, insight, and vision. They were literally named for what I saw—but without the eye. Only the radiating geometry remained. And I couldn't help but wonder: why leave out the eye? Had it been lost over generations? Or was it once too sacred to depict? And then the thought came: what if I had seen the full version?

This realization opened a deeper door. I started tracing the pattern, and it wasn't just Mexico. Identical stepped pyramids rose in both Guatemala and Cambodia—separated by oceans, yet sharing architectural principles, astronomical alignments, and even ceremonial platforms at their summits. Winged sun-disks, nearly indistinguishable in form, adorned temples in both Egypt and Mesopotamia—always hovering above kings and gods, as if to signal their divine right and cosmic origin. Bird-headed figures holding mysterious handbags were carved into stone in ancient Sumeria—and again in the temples and artifacts of Ecuador, their postures and implements eerily consistent. These "handbags" appeared repeatedly beside trees of life, water vessels, or gates—suggesting not tools, but symbols of power, perhaps even devices of transport or transformation. Spiraling, all-seeing symbols watched from Assyrian bas-reliefs and Mesoamerican codices alike—eyes within wheels, suns within squares, sometimes feathered, sometimes winged, always centered. It was the same idea recurring across the globe: an intelligence watching from above, embedded in layered geometries that echoed outward like the rings of reality itself. Sometimes it was a sun. Sometimes a disk. Sometimes a god. Sometimes only the squares. But the shape endured—as if each culture had touched the same memory but carved it in different tongues.

What if these weren't parallel mythologies, but cultural echoes of a shared memory? Not just imagination, but contact? Not coincidence, but convergence? It began to feel as though the winged eye I had seen wasn't unique at all. It was simply remembered differently by different civilizations. Perhaps the Greys had shown it before. And what I witnessed in 1995 was not a symbol created for me... but something ancient, projected again, from a library far older than memory.

4

A LIFE INTERRUPTED

Two years after this incident in my bedroom, I met Nancy, a coworker of mine at Cahner's Publishing. It was on a Friday, June 7th 1996 when after work, a mutual friend of ours named Peggy Anderson invited me to a happy-hour gathering of Cahner's people. The meeting was at a Moretti's restaurant in Edison Park, IL. Known for good pizza, decent Italian fare and a place where one could enjoy a beer with friends, Moretti's was a favorite of our trade-magazine crowd.

That evening, some of the editorial staff for "Restaurants & Institutions" magazine were hanging out - among them, my future wife Nancy. I was from the Graphic Production department, and while I sometimes interacted with sales people from each of the company's numerous magazines, I had never met Nancy - an associate editor. But I knew her coworker, Peggy and trusted her enough to meet up with their group - and be introduced to this captivating woman she told me about.

That evening, Nancy and I got along famously. I was struck by her outgoing, extroverted personality - which seemed to complement my more reserved demeanor. She told me how she was an amateur actor by hobby, performing in local theater plays. She had also previously taken classes and performed at the "Improv Olympic" where she learned from its founder, Del Close - and had the opportunity to interact with comedian Stephen Colbert, who was still involved with "iO" during her time there. As a creative person, I appreciated her own creativity in this medium with which I was unfamiliar. I appreciated her warmth and direct personality - that seemed to operate without much of a social filter. But it was a charming quality that she wore well and it worked for her. Nancy was popular in her circles, as she enjoyed making people laugh. She made every social gathering into a kind of party where she could "perform" to the delight of her friends. The night we met, we traded numbers. We began dating and within a few months were in a serious, committed relationship. I was 27 and she was 33 - just days older than my brother Ron.

Within six months, Nancy and I were engaged. And by October of 1997, we married in a traditional church ceremony surrounded by all our friends and family. Six months before the ceremony we had rented an apartment together in Arlington Heights, IL - one we would share through the time of our wedding and her subsequent pregnancy which began in February of 1998. By October, we had purchased a house in Hoffman Estates, IL and spent a month making it livable before it was time for Nancy to give birth.

In November, we welcomed our daughter, Miranda, into the world. While I was excited and nervous during the labor and birth, something changed within me the moment she arrived. I was overcome with emotion. I cried. My whole being was awash with love, gratitude, and awe. Physically, Miranda was perfect, and she passed the physician's inspection with flying colors—beautiful brown eyes, a lock of brown hair, and the unmistakable glow of health. In the midst of all this, I looked forward to building the foundation of a beautiful future—our home, our daughter, our life together.

In her first twelve months, she was the brightest, happiest child a person could ask for: engaging, curious, and full of life. Right around the age of fourteen months, she was already trying to read her storybooks by flipping the pages and mimicking the way her mother and I would trace our fingers along the words. She would babble syllables like "da da da da," "do do do do," and "ba ba ba ba," mimicking the cadence of speech as if the words were just within her grasp. She was so close to having precocious speech—so close to taking off.

For a while, we did build the life I had dreamed of. But in the blink of an eye, everything changed. In January 2000, both Nancy and Miranda became permanently disabled at the same time, and the life I had envisioned for us collapsed into something unrecognizable.

The previous month, in December of 1999, our 15-month-old daughter Miranda received her scheduled round of pediatric inoculations, including the MMR vaccine (Measles, Mumps, Rubella). At first, we thought nothing of it—it was a routine step, one all parents took. But then Miranda immediately spiked a 105-degree fever that wouldn't break for nearly a week. Her tiny body burned with heat, and when the fever finally subsided, something had changed. She lost her early speech, stopped making eye contact, and developed persistent gastrointestinal issues that doctors struggled to explain. It was like something in her had shut down.

As we scrambled to understand what was happening to our daughter, something equally devastating struck our family. The live measles virus in Miranda's vaccine had shed—a phenomenon I barely understood at the time—and infected Nancy, most likely during a diaper change. What followed was something out of a nightmare.

One day in January, 2000 I had come home from work, entering the front door of our house. As expected, Miranda was running around, playing and Nancy lay on the couch listlessly watching television. At first glance things seemed okay, but then I noticed Miranda had apparently knocked over a potted plant that once rested on our end table. Its dirt was scattered over our new living room rug and the pot and plant itself were separated as they lay on the floor.

Puzzled, I asked Nancy what had happened. She looked at me with a confused expression similar to someone who was inebriated or "high." Nancy looked down at the plant and the dirt on the floor and said simply "Oh, yeah..." her voice trailing off as she made a dismissive wave with her right hand, then reaffixed her gaze to the television.

Standing in the foyer, and trying to understand the scene before me, I asked "Nancy, why didn't you pick up the plant? Why didn't you vacuum? Are you okay?"

"I'm okay," Nancy replied. But clearly she was not okay. I called her brother Joseph on the phone, who lived nearby. After a brief conversation her brother insisted I take her to the emergency room. I agreed.

After her brother and his partner Angelo arrived to babysit Miranda, I drove Nancy to Northwestern Memorial Hospital in Evanston, IL about an hour east of us. Her doctor was there and Northwestern accepted our medical insurance.

During her tests, Nancy was clearly weak and confused. When questioned, She couldn't remember things she had just done. What was worse, she had forgotten we had a child - and that she had given birth to our daughter 16 months previously! It was the year 2000, but she was convinced the year was 1986, a full decade before we had even met. Her words slurred, her thoughts tangled. It was as if I was watching my wife's mind unravel before my eyes.

When the doctors showed me Nancy's MRI scans, my stomach dropped. The image resembled raisin bread—lesions covered every lobe of her brain. The neurologist said it was the worst flare up of Multiple Sclerosis they had ever seen. I stood there in shock, unable to process what I was looking at. "Flare-up," they called it. Flare-up? As if this was something she had always had? But Nancy had seemed perfectly healthy before this. The term made no sense. The doctors didn't have answers, just treatments—plasmapheresis to cleanse her blood and remove the lesions from her brain - and to try and slow the damage.

For a full month, Nancy remained hospitalized at Northwestern. Every night after work, I drove straight to the hospital to be by her side, while my parents took care of Miranda. I was terrified. I needed Nancy. I couldn't do this alone. I remember standing in that cold hospital hallway, my hands trembling, wondering how I was supposed to hold my family together when both my wife and my daughter had been taken from me—one by disease, the other by silence.

When Nancy was finally discharged, she was never the same. Four months later, Miranda was officially diagnosed with "PDD-NOS (Pervasive Developmental Disorder – Not Otherwise Specified), with autism." This meant she was on the autism spectrum but also exhibited severe intellectual disability. Our new family was unraveling before it had even fully begun.

Years of Survival

Over the next seven years, I became both a provider and a caretaker for my wife and daughter. Each year, Nancy's condition worsened, while Miranda continued to grow—bigger, stronger, and harder to handle - given that she was nonverbal, low-functioning and hyperactive.

At first, Nancy still managed to be a stay-at-home mom, taking Miranda to her therapy appointments, even running errands. But by 2005, she started getting lost in the car, even in familiar places. The grocery store, just minutes from our house, had become a maze she couldn't navigate. More than once, she called me from the road, sobbing, panicked, completely disoriented—with Miranda in the backseat.

Each time, I stayed on the phone, my voice steady even as my heart pounded, guiding her home turn by turn like a dispatcher in an emergency. When she finally pulled into the driveway, I would take a deep breath, forcing down the rising panic, knowing it was only going to get worse. By 2006, her ability to drive safely had all but disappeared, forcing me to take her car from her - a decision supported by her family.

Nancy's mother (and sometimes her siblings) helped when they could, hiring a house cleaner and even managing our bills when Nancy could no longer handle finances. But by this point, both Nancy and Miranda suffered from incontinence. After a full day of work, I would come home to clean up after both of them.

Some nights, Miranda would smear the contents of her diaper on the walls, creating what I grimly called fecal frescoes. Other nights, Nancy would have her own accidents. I became an expert at cleaning up poop. So much so that I stopped being disgusted by it—it was just another part of life. But I was exhausted.

By 2008, Nancy's behavior changed drastically. She became belligerent, impatient, erratic—lashing out at me, even in public. She could no longer be trusted alone with Miranda, who was now a flight risk. She would bolt out of the house without warning, with no concept of danger. Sometimes she would run into the busy street. Or leave the house in the middle of winter in her pajamas. And Nancy was too neurologically frail to pursue, or wrangle Miranda when she was being difficult. We hired a home care worker through social services, but it wasn't enough. I was stretched thin between working a full time job, tending to my wife and daughter's special needs while I also handled most of the housekeeping and cooking chores. And worrying about each new crisis that seemed to emerge several times a week.

I started having panic attacks. My hands would go numb, my chest would tighten, and I couldn't breathe. Before I understood these were panic attacks, there was one occasion where I drove to the emergency room for a battery of cardiac tests. There was no hope for the future. No peace at home. No escape. The guilt was unbearable, but after consulting with family, I made the hardest decision of my life. I filed for divorce.

The Fallout

I had hoped Nancy's family would understand. That they would see that I was drowning and couldn't care for them both alone. I needed Nancy's family to take responsibility for her care. And while I was sure they would, I thought I could maintain friendly relations with her family. But instead, her mother waged a war against me.

The divorce dragged on for thirteen months—not because we had anything to fight over, but because Nancy's mother was determined to ensure I was left with nothing. The fight permanently severed our families. When it was over, I never saw any of them again except for Nancy —and neither did Miranda.

That was perhaps the greatest betrayal of all. I had fought to keep some sense of family together, yet in the end, Miranda lost an entire half of her relatives—not by my choice, but by theirs.

Finding Purpose in the Pain

In 2003, while still deep in the trenches of caregiving, I co-founded a nonprofit organization with my friend Julie Duffield, who had two autistic children of her own. Julie and her husband, Joseph were recent transplants from Salt Lake City, Utah. Nancy and I had met the Duffields at our local IHOP restaurant, where we were seated at adjacent tables. We bonded over the obvious similarities in our children's behaviors and similar diagnoses. Joseph and Julie were staying at an Extended Stay America hotel for the next month while their home was being prepared for their move-in date. After we left the restaurant, I prevailed upon Nancy that we should find a way to contact the Duffields at their hotel and invite them to our house for dinner. We did just that! The Duffields were thrilled at the invitation - and thusly began our enduring friendship.

After a few months of our first meeting, Julie Duffield and I were conversing and lamenting how so many medical mysteries plagued our children's health, contributing to their cognitive difficulties. We decided to form a nonprofit so we could help parents find therapies, medical interventions and other resources that their children need. Most parents during these years had difficulty finding answers in those early years of the internet.

Julie and I founded "The Foundation for Autism Information & Research, Inc." aka "FAIR Autism Media." We did some research and found there were a number of biomedical conferences around the country that featured the information and resources we knew parents could use for their children. We decided to raise funds and purchase camera and video production equipment so we could document these resources and disseminate them on the internet.

We traveled the country, attending conferences hosted by "Autism One," the Autism Society of America, and the National Autism Association, filming interviews with doctors, scientists, and parents, and publishing our work for free on our new website — bridging the gap between desperate families and the resources they needed.

At first, I thought I was just helping others. But over time, I realized... I was also saving myself.

Each interview, each conference, each conversation with another heartbroken parent reminded me: I wasn't alone. I wasn't the only one who had lost the life they had envisioned. And if I couldn't fix what had happened to my own family, at least I could make it mean something.

For ten years, this mission gave me a reason to keep going. But by 2013, the weight of single fatherhood became too much to maintain extracurricular responsibilities. I passed control of the foundation to our board chairman in New York, Michael Smith, and life carried on.

But the grief never left me. I had dreamed of a full family. Of raising multiple children and being the kind of father I was blessed to have. Instead, disease took everything.

For years, my focus had been on survival—caring for Miranda, keeping myself afloat, and trying to make sense of the wreckage that disease had left behind. The strange experiences I had in childhood and the incident in 1994 weren't of the slightest concern in my life — none of it mattered in the face of more pressing concerns, nor did I have the slightest reason to give those memories a revisit. My world was grounded in earthly struggles—family, caretaking and survival.

Single Parenting and Autism

The weight of single parenthood was unlike anything I had ever known. While most people went home from work to rest or unwind, I came home to a second shift—one filled with caretaking, crisis management, and an ever-present hum of anxiety. Miranda required constant attention. After she came home from school, she couldn't be left alone for even a few minutes. For a time, I was fortunate to have home care workers assigned through social services—young women who would arrive shortly before her school bus dropped her off. They'd retrieve her, help her settle in, and stay with her until I returned from work. On paper, it was a manageable plan. In reality, it was full of holes.

Caregivers called in sick all the time. Or quit with little notice. Some were no-shows, and I'd only find out when the school bus arrived at my driveway with no one there to meet it. On those days, I'd have to leave work in a panic—embarrassed, apologetic, scrambling to beat the clock. I knew my boss had limits. And every last-minute excuse chipped away at their patience. There were no backup systems, no safety net. Just me.

The stress was relentless. I worried not just about Miranda's daily needs, but about my job, my ability to keep a roof over our heads, and what would happen if I ever got sick or injured. I didn't have the luxury of falling apart. There was no partner to lean on, no family member who could take over. I had to stay standing.

I tried dating during those years. At first, I thought it might be possible to find companionship again—to rebuild something of a normal life. I met women on dating sites, and many of them were kind and receptive to meeting me for dinner. But when the conversation turned to my home life—to Miranda's condition, her level of disability, the demands of raising her alone—I could see the air go out of their expression. They weren't unkind about it, just honest. Most of them quietly moved on.

Even my friends started to fade. I was always declining invitations —to parties, to dinners, to weekend get-togethers—because I never had coverage. After a while, the invitations stopped coming. I understood. People had their own lives. But it left me deeply isolated. My world was small, bounded by work and caretaking, with little time left for anything else. And not many people really understood what my life looked like on the inside.

But it wasn't all hardship. There were moments, even amid the stress and exhaustion, that felt like grace. When the house was quiet, and Miranda sat peacefully on the couch with her iPad—lost in the joy of her music—I would pause whatever I was doing just to watch her. Her fingers moved delicately across the screen, her eyes locked in focus, her expression calm. Sometimes she would smile to herself, and I would just... ache. She looked so beautiful in her serenity. All my work, all my effort—it was to provide for moments like this.

Other times, when she'd grow tired of her music, she would walk over to me, climb into my lap, and rest her head on my shoulder. It always took me by surprise. It felt like an angel had chosen to land—not with words, but with presence. She didn't need to speak. Her love was unmistakable and perfect.

And there were our walks—always at our local park in Hoffman Estates. Fabbrini Park is a large, beautiful and well-appointed suburban oasis that provides its locals with a variety of amenities: playground equipment, tennis courts, baseball diamonds and soccer fields. But also a lovely, paved walking path that meandered around and between two man-made lakes that reflect the sky, with willow trees that bow gently toward the water. Large birds such as ducks, geese, egrets and cranes would often grace their waters. We'd stroll the curved path together, often in silence, sometimes hand-in-hand. Miranda loved the swing sets, the wildlife, the wind. And I loved those moments. They were quiet and ordinary and everything.

Those were the moments that kept me going.

For years, this was the essence of my existence. Rooted in routine and grounded by necessity, my life looked nothing like the reality that was looming on the horizon. The stark contrast between the myopic concerns of parenthood and the cosmic revelations that crept in from the shadows could not have been more different or more jarring. But despite that contrast and my attempts to examine it, the divisions were grey and vague - and my life would be filled with the angst of unanswerable questions to come.

5

THROUGH OPEN EYES

Twenty six years after the incident where I saw the greys in my apartment bedroom, I was a stay at home, single father raising my profoundly autistic daughter during the COVID pandemic. Her school had already been shut down for several months, and very few services for childcare existed to aid me and my ability to work. So I found myself working freelance projects in graphic design and renting out spare bedrooms via Airbnb to make ends meet.

In early March of 2020, I began to notice unusual things happening in my bedroom between when I'd go to sleep at night and when I'd awaken in the morning. Among the first of these was that, upon waking, I noticed my bed's comforter was oriented ninety degrees the wrong way, as the bedding was adorned with large gold and black stripes. This was unusual because, even on my roughest of nights where I may toss and turn, I never shifted my bedding by a full ninety degrees. Not even once. To make this change even more perplexing, I noticed that my bamboo backscratcher and sleep mask, which usually sit atop the comforter, were now neatly placed beside me under my top sheet.

These two accessories usually get kicked off the bed during a rough night. So if I were to assume that the previous night was fitful, I'd expect the backscratcher and sleep mask to be on the floor on the opposite side of the bed. But here they were, beside me. Under the top sheet. And I know my nature. I wouldn't have placed them there. Simply because I don't want to roll on top of a piece of bamboo with a sharp-ish end that could wake me up. So when I awoke to the repositioned comforter, it was notable for me. It didn't, however, mean anything in and of itself.

Another incident that startled me involved some ear plugs that I would wear at night to help block out extraneous noise from the hallway, or from the street. As an AirBnB host, I would regularly be awakened by my guests who open and close the bathroom door across the hall from my room. On the night in question, I went to bed with the soft foam earplugs in my ear canals and fell into a restful sleep. When I awoke the next morning, I could feel that I wasn't wearing the earplugs.

"Oh, I must have taken them out and didn't remember" I thought. As I turned to check my dresser, which I use as a nightstand, I expected to see the ear plugs where I would always toss them, atop the dresser somewhere next to the white noise machine or candle holders. They would be laying on their sides, probably four inches apart from one another and possibly one of them would have rolled off the dresser to land on my bedroom's shag carpeting. But that wasn't the case. As expected, I found the earplugs, but they were neatly placed. Rather daintily and politely on their ends, side by side.

Nobody but myself would have found that disturbing. But as I said, I know my nature. I did not place the earplugs on the nightstand so neatly. Nor did I rotate my own bedding a full ninety degrees in that previous occurrence.

These two incidents alone would have caused me to ask questions, but there were a few more as this was occurring every four to six weeks, roughly. Collectively, they were demanding my attention. Since I am single and lived alone save for my daughter in the next room, there was no one else to which I could attribute small changes in my bedroom environment. And I could safely rule out being pranked by my AirBnB guests, as they were short term renters and never entered my room.

I had to assume that these incidents were attributable to something OTHER than any people I'm aware of, including my guests, my daughter or myself. Somewhere deep in my mind was that twenty six year old memory of the four small greys whooshing out of my apartment bedroom in 1994. That seemingly one-off incident that, without evidence or proof, was dismissed as a fading memory as the years advanced. Could these disturbances in my room be THEM? As a question, or idea, it was as eccentric as you can get. Despite that, by mid April I had decided to conduct a simple experiment - one for which I had low expectations.

The Sign

"Once you eliminate the impossible, whatever remains, no matter how improbable, must be the truth." -Arthur Conan Doyle

It occurred to me that if I were to determine whether alien, grey beings were disturbing me in my bedroom as I slept, I'd need to communicate with them. Hypothetically, given the assumption I couldn't wake myself to do so during their visit(s), I'd have to leave a sign on the wall and hope they can read English. So that's what I decided to do.

The next evening, I searched google images for an illustration of a grey alien. I Found one that resembled what I saw 26 years earlier and placed it prominently on a small poster with large, block letters that stated "I WANT TO REMEMBER YOUR VISIT. LET ME REMEMBER YOU. I WILL NOT HARM." Simple, and to the point. I printed out the poster on my iMac and taped it to the wall above my headboard. Seeing the sign taped to the wall, I couldn't help feeling self conscious. "Do I really believe this is a possibility?" I hoped nobody would enter my room, see the sign and think I needed psychiatric help. They would be forgiven for thinking so. It's a little nuts. Most likely, however, nothing would happen, and after a time I'll take the sign down, clean the tape smudge off the paint and toss the poster in the trash. And my unanswered curiosity would remain a mystery.

Confirmation, however, proved itself a much bigger mystery.

After about a week had gone by, I had grown accustomed to having that sign above my bed. No longer feeling self conscious about it, the poster just hung there night after night. I had become busy with my daily routines, managing my freelance graphic design work, taking care of my airbnb rooms and the needs of my autistic daughter. "Real Life" had interceded and my little experiment had already begun to bore me. But there was no reason to take the sign down yet. A second week would pass without incident. It was now the end of the last week of April, 2020.

Then, one night - like an unexpected slap in the face, I awoke suddenly around 3:00 a.m. or a little after, in my garage. I can only guess the time. I was mostly naked, save for the briefs I wear to bed, paralyzed and suspended off my feet above the garage floor. I could feel very little other than the lack of warmth in the garage but I was very conscious as my body was tilted forward to afford me the very clear view of a small grey alien before me, about six feet away. He was dressed in black coveralls from neck to foot, staring up at me. While I couldn't move my body, I was able to move my head. To my left was my red 2002 Chevy Trailblazer and to my right, the side door of the garage, granting access to the back yard. The Grey was a little more than three and a half feet tall. Small, thin and frail in appearance. Yet it was in complete control of my five-foot-ten, 220 pound body as I floated light as a feather above the concrete floor.

The Grey was standing adjacent to the garage's side window which itself was next to the side door. He was illuminated by very bright, streaming white light that came through the window and seemed to dance side-to-side as to suggest a moving light source. Without it, the garage would have been totally dark.

As I hung there, helpless, I took in the sight before me with stunned awe. If I had been allowed to speak, I wouldn't have anything to communicate. I was in a state of awareness and suppressed shock. Numbed both physically and emotionally. After five to seven seconds, the Grey spoke to me placing words in my mind... in english. "We can't allow you to remember our visit, because my superiors will know about it." I was conscious for two to three seconds more, trying to comprehend what was happening and what its words meant. Before I could formulate a question, I was unconscious again and woke up back in my bed. I sat up and looked at the clock that sits atop a shelf on the adjacent wall. It was 3:35 a.m.

Was I asleep for awhile after they returned me? Or did I awaken immediately after? I can't be certain, which is why I had to guess what time I awoke in the garage. Physically, I felt perfectly okay. I didn't feel traumatized. I could liken it to being intoxicated during the experience. As though they have a way to suppress your nervous system so your memories won't impress upon you as deeply and give you license to dismiss what occurred as some kind of vivid dream. But this was no dream. I know what my dreams are like and I know what being awake in my garage is like. Also, my visual memory is very strong. I'm a graphic designer and art director. I think visually and I recall everything visually. At no point did I suspect or dismiss what happened as a dream. And that forces me to contemplate the profundity of what occurred.

I had just seen a small, grey alien creature that resembled the four I witnessed 26 years earlier, who whooshed out of my bedroom. Saying it again, I had just seen a small, grey alien creature! Which means what happened in 1994 was not only real, it wasn't a random occurrence. These things are here for ME. Why? What does any of this mean? Should I have assumed they would return?

Meet My Superior

I spent the following week as I did most weeks that first year of COVID, tending to my daughter, cleaning my rental rooms and I greeted a few traveling nurses as guests. But in the back of my mind was the specter of what had just happened. I didn't know how to feel about it and I certainly didn't know what to "do" about it. I hesitated to tell anyone what had happened. My real fear was that those who know me will recall times in my childhood when I was extremely imaginative and enjoyed playing "pretend" games. Not that they wouldn't trust my sincerity, but could they trust my judgment? Without witnesses, how do you pull out this story that is beyond any experiential frame of reference and just plop it in front of them? Sure, most people I know probably have watched Hollywood movies and TV shows dealing with the subject of alien visitors and UFO's, etcetera, but it's quite a leap to ask anyone to internalize it. To personalize it. "Hey mom, your baby boy is being kidnapped at night by aliens!" What do you say to that? What do you expect anyone to say to that?

Setting aside my fear of speaking about the matter, I was quite curious, albeit apprehensive about any future encounters. Would there be another one? Or would I have to wait 26 years before the next one? The answer to that question presented itself sooner than I could have expected.

After a week had passed since the garage encounter, I awoke suddenly because of sounds of movement and the physical sensation of something brushing across my comforter, atop my legs. My eyes popped open and they were met with another pair of eyes, five inches from my face! There in my vision was another alien. Its face had large black eyes that wrapped around the corner of its temples, a nearly flat nose with slits and a small mouth. It had elephant-grey skin that resembled unpolished leather and I could see not only its face, but its chest and shoulders, which weren't clothed. This creature was not like the others. Instantly I could estimate it as taller than the little ones that had been in my bedroom 26 years earlier, or the one in the garage.

"He" was partially laying on me. His feet were making contact with the bed and he appeared to have both hands on either side of me, propping his upper torso at an angle so as to place our faces at mutual eye level.

His eyes were a deep black with slight glossy highlights at the edges. While the room was dark, there was illumination between the two of us, with no discernible source of light. And this light was just adequate to allow me to see three smaller greys in my periphery, standing to my right beside the bed. They were shadowed, but visible.

As He moved his face closer to mine, I felt the sense that I was meant to look directly into his eyes. As I was too intimidated to do so, I found myself observing his right shoulder while I avoided his gaze. I began to notice the texture of his skin. I was completely paralyzed, but upon his noticing that I was inspecting his shoulder, he seemed to know that I wanted to touch him. Quite suddenly, I was able to move my left arm. But only my left arm. I raised my left hand and maneuvered it into the tight space between our chests. I gently placed my fingertips on the top of his right shoulder as my thumb grasped the area of his collarbone. I gripped his shoulder as I dragged my fingertips over the grey, leather like skin. It reminded me a little like elephant skin, but its texture was tighter and smoother. The shoulder had almost zero subcutaneous fat. It was very tight, sinewy and bony. After a few moments of this, my level of apprehension had subsided and I felt comfortable enough to raise my eyes to his. What did he want? Why are they back?

As our eyes met for a more sustained gaze, he moved his face closer and touched his forehead to mine. It was at this moment that I instantly fell unconscious and into a lucid dreaming state. This was the kind of dream where you are aware that you're asleep and understand that the images you see aren't reality. And yet, this would be the most real lucid dream I'd ever experienced. Because it was given to me. It was induced.

As suddenly as I lost consciousness, I found myself in this dream state, standing on a slightly sloped, cobblestone street. Below us about 200 feet away was a Bavarian style building in half-timbered architecture. And further down that street, I could see more buildings in that style. Distinctive brown timbered framework, criss-crossed with white stuccoed plaster between the timbers. Was this meant to resemble Germany?

The sky above us was lit by a full moon, which seemed fitting, because it was the end of the first week of May, 2020 and we did in fact have a full moon.

In front of me was the tall, darker skinned grey, whose shoulder I was inspecting just a moment ago. Like me, he stood on the cobblestone street and behind him was a grassy slope with a stone stair passage up the hill from the street we were standing on. And to my right were three identical little girls, all the same height with blue eyes and blonde hair, all wearing the same dresses. Or at least that's how I was supposed to see them.

The "tall" grey was about five feet two inches in height. The girls matched the height of the short greys I've seen which were about 42 inches, or 3 feet six inches. I found myself able to ask the tall grey questions, and for some reason, felt the need to "translate" the telepathy I was having with him by speaking verbally to the little girls. At the time, I was seduced into believing they were little girls, and not the three greys in my bedroom, accompanying this tall grey.

"What's your name?" I asked the tall grey.

"Syczilick," he replied with his answer ringing clearly in my mind. He made no audible sounds.

I turned to the little girls and knelt down slightly in front of them to repeat his reply to me.

"He said his name is Syczilick... or Syliczyk." I wasn't certain I was pronouncing it correctly. The three girls stared blankly at me.

"Are you from Zeta 2 Reticuli?" I asked next, as I stood and turned back toward him. This question popped into my mind, as I was previously familiar with the Betty and Barney Hill abduction story. My whole life I had an unexplainable interest in UFO's and abductions, so began reading more on the subject in the mid 1990's, after my 1994 bedroom encounter. In the Betty and Barney Hill abduction, it was Betty who recalled being shown a star map that related the position of our sun to their own solar system. Some time after Betty shared her star map, redrawn during hypnotic memory regression, a school teacher and amateur astronomer named Marjorie Fish was able to correlate the map to stars visible from the southern hemisphere.

"Yes," he replied. They were from Zeta 2 Reticuli.

"And Is your planet named Serpo?" Again, my question came from things I had read, this time a briefing paper alleged to have been shared with President Ronald Reagan after his first inauguration. The military, it seems, calls the home world of these greys "Serpo." If the Reagan briefing memo is to be believed.

"No," he answered. "We don't call it that."

I waited briefly, hoping he would volunteer their own name for their world, but this "Syczilick" was more of a 'yes-or-no' speaker. Nothing volunteered. Strictly business. Honestly, I was lucky to have this type of encounter and the ability to ask questions. I wish I had thought of better questions. But I was fighting confusion in the midst of this induced dream environment.

As before, I knelt down to tell the little girls that the Grey named "Syczilick" didn't call his planet "Serpo."

Just then, the little girl in the middle looked me squarely in the eyes and exclaimed "You know? You're nice. We were told you would be mean."

Her words took me aback a moment. "Mean?" Why would someone tell them that I am a mean person? Before I could formulate that question to ask them, the induced dream had ended. Everything went black.

I awoke some time after they had left. Looking around my room, they were no longer there. The clock read 3:45 a.m. Just then, I heard my autistic daughter Miranda, giggling in her bedroom next to mine. We shared a wall. I jumped out of bed to go check on her, my first thought being "Are they bothering her too?" If they were, I was going to confront them! But it could otherwise be that she wet her pull-up garment and needed changed. I entered her room, which was illuminated by the setting full moon shining through her mini blinds. She was alone, thank God. Checking her pull-up garment, I noticed it was dry. She only wakes up when she's wet. What's going on? Had they been entertaining her while messing with her daddy? As she is nonverbal, she couldn't tell me such things. I may never know.

After verifying my daughter was okay, I left Miranda's room and did a walking tour of the house, wanting to be sure these "people" were truly gone. After returning to my bedroom, my thoughts turned to what had just happened. I had to process all of this. It occurred to me that I am being visited by two kinds of creatures that have masterful control over my body and my mind. What was this taller grey about? Was he one of the "superiors" alluded to by the little grey in my garage the previous week? Was he there to investigate how I discovered they were 'visiting' me? By using that sign on my wall, I was bluffing. I had nothing to go on, but a 26 year old vague memory of little white headed people zipping out of my bedroom. And now I realize that the little one that pulled me to the side in my garage for a private chat, may have been breaking protocol.

I can imagine that despite their carefulness each time they were coming for me and keeping me unconscious for whatever the hell they were doing, I somehow figured them out and they were baffled, if not startled, by my sign. Perhaps the little one that took me into the garage before returning me to my bedroom was hoping to learn something. But didn't. And that's why "Syczylick" came to check me out.

Perhaps in some suppressed memory, I might have been asked questions by Syczylick. Perhaps he learned that his little workers were sloppy in previous visits and I was smart enough to piece the clues together? I wish I could find out.

The Visits Become Routine

As 2020 progressed, I had five or six more visits in my room that caught my attention. After Syczilick's visit, my wait was only six weeks before I would see these greys again. In the wee hours of Friday morning of June 19th, 2020 I awoke to the sounds and sensations of movement in my room, despite the comforting rush of whooshing air circulating inside my white noise machine on the dresser. Startled at these sensations, I opened my eyes to a darkened room, the only illumination offered by the red numbers of my alarm clock on the opposite wall. I couldn't move my body but was able to move my head a little. I noticed two individuals standing to my right, completely shadowed by the dark room, but discernible as my eyes adjusted their focus. As I noticed them, sounds to my left alerted me to the presence of two others on the opposite side of my bed. "They're HERE" was the only thought that entered my mind.

Just then, two of the individuals from both sides of the bed traded positions, by lifting off the ground and criss-crossing one another above me as they levitated to their new spots. I was struggling to stay awake and focus my eyes, but as they were crossing paths above my body, I noticed these two individuals had a light green aurora ever so slightly outlining the edges of their bodies. This aurora also allowed me to see their faces, which seemed to be grinning at me. I was awake for a total of 10 or 12 seconds. Once these two little greys had changed positions around my bed, I fell unconscious. Whatever transpired during their visit, I can only guess.

When I awoke again as the rising sun shone through the gaps in my window curtains, I noticed that my right ear canal was in pain, as though a large object had been inserted and stretched the opening for too long. I sat up in bed, feeling my right ear and exploring the opening with my index finger. "Do I have an earache? Or did these things insert something in my ear?" This was to be the first of physical aftereffects I would experience in subsequent encounters. But it reminded me of one of the first clues I had of their visits, when my earplugs had been removed and carefully placed on the dresser. What's with my right ear? Are they using something in my ear to subdue me? Also, WHY are they visiting me? What are they doing when they have me paralyzed? The answer to that last question would present itself with their very next visit.

During the next six weeks, I spent my time on matters of childcare, trying to see if I could secure more hours for my daughter's in-home personal care assistant, Cathi. The more hours I could secure, I'd be able to spend on freelance graphic design projects that were supplementing my AirBnB income, in addition to my daughter's SSI payments. And as it was summer, my daughter and I spent a number of hours each nice day walking at a nearby park. Miranda loves the peaceful surroundings of the walking path as it meanders around two artificial lakes and their visiting wildlife. And I found the park's tranquil nature to be therapeutic. The long walks and the fact that my daughter was nonverbal, allowed me to quietly reflect on the esoteric matters with which I was being confronted.

On July 29th, 2020 I had another in-home encounter that gave me insight on what they do during their visits. As before, I'd awaken as a result of movement sensations and errant sounds disturbing the monotone static of my white noise machine. But this time, as I opened my eyes, I became aware of the sensation of my top sheet and comforter being pulled downward, off my legs. Before I had gained my bearings, my first instinct was to reach down and catch my sheets before they could hit the floor at the foot of the bed. In my mind and at that moment, they were merely sliding off the bed… despite the fact that they never do that. But I couldn't move. I couldn't react to the sheets coming off my body and I felt the cooler air of the room spill onto my skin. The room, this time, was illuminated with a soft pale green light, the source of which I couldn't see.

In my confused state, I hadn't yet thought I was being visited again, but perplexed why I couldn't move. However as I was gaining clarity in the span of several seconds, I also felt someone's hands and fingers insert themselves between my underwear briefs and my hips, followed by my briefs sliding down my legs. And I could feel finger tips hitting my calves as the briefs were being removed. It happened so quickly that by the time I had tilted my head forward and moved my eyes downward toward my feet to see who was doing this, the briefs were already off and I saw my visitors.

There were four small greys. Three to my right at the edge of the bed and one at its foot, who was now placing my bunched up briefs on the bed's fitted sheet, to the left corner.

I was naked. I felt as though I should be panicking but I was strangely calm, as my emotional response was as muted as the sensations I was experiencing. I could FEEL the removal of the sheets and my underwear, and I could feel the air was cooler, but it was definitely muted. I did not have full access to all my senses. And I couldn't understand how I was feeling. I should be jumping out of the bed, picking these little fuckers up off the ground and throwing them against the wall, as would a startled person brush off and crush a spider. But it wasn't like that at all and I find that confusing.

Just then, as I was still conscious and looking at the grey at the foot of the bed, I felt my mind become cloudy as the grey's face seemed to morph into the face of an unattractive woman I know. What the hell? The grey, now in the mental guise of this homely woman I would never choose, crawled over the foot of the bed and over my legs, staring into my eyes the entire time. "Would you like a blow job?" this "woman" asked me. In my entranced confusion I found myself believing to be alone with a woman and I felt my penis begin to erect itself. "Sure," I said, bewildered. At that moment, the face before me feigned a movement as though "she" were going to perform fellatio, but at the last second pulled her face away and with her right hand placed a device over my genitals. I got a quick glance of the device before I lost consciousness. It was shaped at the large opening like an athletic cup... somewhat of a curved triangle, and converges to a point like a smoothed three sided cone. And it was colored black.

I was only conscious for two seconds after the cone had been placed over my genitalia. I don't remember the sensation of climaxing, but sometime after I had awakened, I realized my penis felt sore as it would after a prolonged love-making session. Though at that time, I wasn't presently dating anyone and thusly was not sexually active.

As I mentioned before, this visit would answer one of my questions; "what are they doing here?" It was obvious to me now that they were collecting a semen sample from me. Is that what they always do? Is that why four greys had been in my apartment bedroom in 1994? What are they doing with my semen? I was hoping to discover the answer.

Throughout the remainder of 2020, the visits continued on a four to six week schedule. Not so reliable where I could predict them on a calendar, but they were regular enough that when the next timeframe approached, I'd find myself wondering " is tonight the night?"

Sometimes I'd be conscious for a few seconds and get a glimpse of the little greys. I remember one night in particular where disturbances in my room woke me up and I was laying on my right side, facing my dresser and closet, but my face was buried in a pillow save for my left eye. Upon awakening, there was a light above my head and in my peripheral vision, I saw two hands with long spindly fingers coming toward my head the second before I fell unconscious again.

On a few occasions I would awaken after 3:00 a.m. talking midsentence. "No, I don't want you to visit me tonight!" And I spoke it somewhat loudly. I was not dreaming prior to waking up when I said this. It was deep sleep where everything is black. No REM sleep or dream sequences. I'd wake up from deep sleep saying those words. And my heart was beating faster than normal. I had wondered if I had been taken and recently returned moments before awakening to say those words.

6

UNDER THE SKIN

Sometime in the second week of March, 2021, I woke to the distinct sensation of hands on my body—fingers pressing firmly into my right forearm and bicep. The touch was clinical, controlled, and unmistakably not mine. My eyes opened slowly, and the first thing I saw were four tall greys standing directly over me, all of them staring into my eyes with that unwavering, unreadable stillness they carry like a second skin.

But I wasn't in my bed. I wasn't even in my house.

The surroundings were dim—oppressively so. Only a soft, ambient glow seemed to emanate from nowhere in particular, casting light just far enough to reveal the area around the metallic table I was lying on. The walls, if there were walls, faded into darkness. I had the distinct sense that space itself ended just beyond the halo of light. It was like being suspended in a pocket reality—one made solely for this moment.

Two of the greys were on my right. One stood at my feet. The fourth remained on my left, close enough that I could feel its presence more than see it. I was paralyzed, as I often was in these encounters—my body unresponsive save for my head, which I could turn slightly. Even that small freedom felt like a concession. It was enough to let me see them, but not enough to let me move.

My breath was shallow. My thoughts sluggish, like they were swimming through static. Still, something inside me recognized the familiarity of this scenario. Not the room, not the layout—those were new. But the feeling—the cold stillness, the presence of minds far older than mine—was all too familiar.

The grey at the foot of the table raised a small object into view and held it deliberately, as if to ensure I saw it. In that moment, my mind conjured a bizarre association: the object looked like an old-fashioned vacuum tube, the kind you'd see in a 1950s television or radio. Transparent, cylindrical, with internal components I couldn't quite define. It didn't glow, didn't hum—but it felt alive in a way I can't explain.

Then came the voice. Not audible, but insistent. A thought placed directly into my mind with unsettling clarity: "We are giving you a new one. Be careful with this one, or we won't be able to find you."

A new one? My mind strained to process the words, still crawling out of whatever hypnotic fog had been wrapped around my consciousness. And yet, even through the confusion, I understood. They were showing me an implant. Somehow, I knew it was destined for my abdomen. I didn't need to be told—there was a clarity to the information that bypassed language altogether.

And then—blackness. I awoke back in my room with the time on my clock showing 3:40 a.m.

Their words lingered in my mind long after I woke up. "We are giving you a new one. Be careful with this one, or we won't be able to find you."

It wasn't just an observation—it was a warning. Be careful with this one. What had happened to the old one? Had I somehow lost or damaged a previous implant? Had they been tracking me before with a different device, one that had malfunctioned or been removed? And if they couldn't "find me" without it, what did that imply about its function?

The idea that this implant was necessary for them to locate me suggested something far more advanced than a simple biological monitor. This wasn't just a passive device collecting data. It was actively transmitting my position.

But what else did it do?

In my research, I had heard of abductees discovering small metallic or biological anomalies embedded in their bodies—tiny foreign objects under the skin, often in the ear, nasal cavity, leg, or hand.

Some individuals who had undergone medical imaging or minor surgeries reported doctors finding unusual objects that should not have been there, sometimes encased in fibrous tissue, as though their bodies had attempted to isolate them.

Dr. Roger Leir, a podiatric surgeon who specialized in the removal and analysis of alleged alien implants, spent years studying these objects. According to Leir, some of the implants extracted from abductees contained nano-structured metals, isotopic ratios not found in Earthly materials, and unusual electromagnetic properties. One implant was even reported to have been emitting radio frequencies at 14.7 MHz, suggesting an active transmission capability.

But what truly set his work apart were the cases where biological responses to the implants defied medical explanation. In multiple surgeries, Leir noted that the implants were often found embedded near nerve clusters, and yet the surrounding tissue showed no inflammatory response—as though the body didn't recognize the object as foreign.

In fact, in several cases, the implants were surrounded by what appeared to be neural fibers growing into or around the object itself. Leir's team speculated that this could indicate a kind of bio-integration—a deliberate merging of alien material with human physiology.

In one particularly strange case, an implant removed from a man's leg was found to be coated in a dark, membrane-like sheath that closely resembled keratinized biological tissue, even though the implant underneath was metallic. The sheath was never conclusively identified, but under microscopy, it exhibited properties unlike any known human biological covering. Leir noted that this biological camouflage might be an intentional adaptation—either to avoid detection or to stabilize the object within the host's body over time.

Equally bizarre was the way some of the implants seemed to move or migrate within the body. One subject had an object in his arm that shifted position between scans—appearing at one location during an X-ray, and then at a slightly different depth days later.

Leir and his team tried to explain it away as imaging error, but the pattern repeated itself across multiple subjects. Whether by design or unknown interaction with the body's tissues, some implants appeared to be active even in their dormant state.

Were these implants simply tracking devices, or did they have a more complex role?

The Broader Phenomenon of Alien Implants

The concept of implants placed within abductees is not a new one. Reports of small, foreign objects discovered inside the body without any memory of how they got there have been documented for decades. Often, these implants are found in highly specific locations—the nasal cavity, behind the ear, inside the hand or leg, and sometimes within bone tissue itself. What's more, abductees frequently report feeling nothing during implantation, only discovering them later through X-rays, MRIs, or unexplained wounds that heal unusually fast.

Documented Cases of Alleged Implants

Among the most compelling aspects of the abduction phenomenon are the physical traces left behind—specifically, the implants. Dr. Roger Leir's work is perhaps the most well-known in this arena. He performed over a dozen removals of alleged implants, many of which contained exotic materials. In some cases, the implants were composed of carbon nanotube structures, and a number of them emitted measurable electromagnetic frequencies once removed from the body.

Whitley Strieber also reported his own experiences with implants, most notably in his books *Communion* and *Confirmation*. He described persistent nasal pain, which he attributed to an implant that later seemed to vanish without explanation. But perhaps more disturbingly, in 1998 he experienced something much more direct—a physical sensation of something being inserted into his earlobe. He was fully awake and conscious during the event, describing a sharp, sudden pain and an audible "click" as the object was embedded beneath the skin. A small metallic nodule remained afterward. When a doctor later examined the area, he discovered an unidentifiable foreign body, lending further weight to the experience. Strieber speculated that the device might have been a tracker—or possibly an interface for telepathic communication.

Researcher Derrel Sims also collected numerous reports from abductees who remembered glowing objects embedded beneath their skin. These were not vague memories, but vivid accounts of blue and green luminescent materials seen during or after encounters. Sims' work raised further questions about the variety and possible functions of these implants.

In some of the most frustrating cases, abductees who scheduled surgeries to have implants removed reported that the objects had vanished just before the procedure. Dr. Roger Leir himself documented several of these cases. In *The Aliens and the Scalpel*, he described a patient named "John Smith" (a pseudonym) who had a metallic anomaly in his left toe confirmed by multiple X-rays and a CT scan. The object appeared consistent in shape and location over the course of nearly six months. But when the final pre-operative scan was performed, it was simply gone. No surgical entry, no mark, no residual tissue damage—just an empty space where something undeniably had been.

Another case involved a woman named Pat Parrinellie, who had a visible, palpable lump in her shin that could be felt just beneath the skin. According to Leir, the object was verified with imaging and scheduled for removal—but a few days before the procedure, she awoke with a small, triangular red mark on her leg. When she arrived at the clinic, the object was no longer detectable on touch or scan. The surgery was canceled. In her own words, she felt as though she'd been "visited again to clean up a mess they didn't want left behind."

These weren't isolated anomalies. Researcher Derrel Sims has also documented numerous instances of implants relocating or disappearing entirely. In one of his investigations, an abductee had an object in her arm that moved several centimeters between imaging sessions conducted only days apart. The patient was baffled—and understandably paranoid. Sims noted that in many such cases, abductees report unusual dreams or fragmented memories in the nights leading up to the disappearance. It's as if the object was retrieved during another encounter, or perhaps remotely disabled and dissolved by design.

What disturbed many of these abductees wasn't just the loss of the object—it was the loss of proof. For individuals desperate to validate their experiences—not only to others, but to themselves—the disappearance of an implant felt like being robbed twice: first of bodily autonomy, and then of the one piece of evidence that might have confirmed their reality.

The implications are chilling. If these implants can be removed, relocated, or deactivated without warning, it suggests an active and ongoing surveillance architecture. The technology isn't static—it's responsive. It can evade scrutiny. And that means the control doesn't end when the encounter does. Some abductees have even speculated that implants may be part of a biological leasing system—used for specific phases or data collection periods, then retracted or upgraded.

It raises uncomfortable questions: How many people have carried implants without ever knowing? And how many have unknowingly had them taken back?

The big question, of course, is why? If these implants are simply tracking devices, why place them in so many different areas of the body? Why the variety in composition and function? Some researchers have speculated that the implants may serve multiple purposes—monitoring physiology, recording neurological activity, or even influencing perception and behavior. Others believe that some implants could function as biological cameras, recording sensory information from the abductee's perspective and transmitting it back to their observers.

After my encounter in March 2021, I never felt or found an implant in my abdomen. But that doesn't mean it isn't there. Unlike the more commonly reported subdermal implants—those that can be felt beneath the skin or discovered through casual examination—this one may have been placed deeper inside my body. It could reside in tissue or bone, far beyond my ability to detect without the aid of advanced medical imaging.

If the implant's purpose is to ensure that they can locate me, then what happens if it fails? Are there other abductees who were once part of this program but have since become untraceable—perhaps because their implants were lost or removed? Have some individuals slipped through the cracks, inadvertently abandoned by their captors?

That memory remains vivid—the words still echoing in my mind: "Be careful with this one, or we won't be able to find you." Whatever its purpose, that statement confirms they had been tracking me. If the greys did implant something in me, then in theory, modern imaging technologies should be able to detect it. The question is—which technology would be most effective?

X-rays are the most obvious first step. They're especially good at detecting metallic objects embedded in bone, such as my upper arm's humerus, where I suspect an implant may have been placed. Many abductees have stumbled upon foreign objects this way—during routine dental or orthopedic X-rays.

For soft tissue, an MRI scan might be more appropriate, especially if the implant is composed of non-metallic or biological materials. MRIs can sometimes reveal unusual shapes or densities in tissue that would otherwise go unnoticed.

Ultrasound may also be of use, particularly if the implant is encapsulated in fibrous tissue, which has been reported in a few of Dr. Leir's extracted specimens. The high-frequency waves can sometimes highlight foreign bodies missed by other methods.

Another option is an RF frequency scan. Dr. Leir and others have noted that some implants emit low-level radio frequencies. In theory, a simple handheld RF detector could pick up transmissions if the implant is actively broadcasting—though not all implants may be "on" at any given time.

And then there's the biggest question of all—what happens if I do find something? Would a doctor believe me if I told them the truth about how it got there? Would they be willing to remove it? Or would the object vanish before I had the chance, as has happened in so many other cases?

To this day, I've noticed no physiological changes—no pain, no sensation, no obvious disruption to my biology. Whatever this thing is, it operates in silence. That silence, in its own way, is part of the violation. There's no warning, no aftereffect, no way to prove what's been done unless the implant chooses to reveal itself. It exists in that liminal space—present but hidden, active but undetectable. And maybe that's the point. The perfect monitoring system doesn't announce itself. It simply becomes part of you.

I was beginning to understand that this wasn't just about control or surveillance. It was about erosion. Little by little, they were wearing me down—getting under my skin in more ways than one. These devices weren't merely tools of technology; they were symbolic of something more invasive. My body was no longer mine alone. Every time I tried to reclaim some sense of normalcy, there was always the looming awareness that something foreign might be embedded inside me, transmitting data, overriding boundaries I never consented to cross. It wasn't just physical. It was psychological. Existential. They weren't just inside my body. They were inside my life.

I don't know the answers. But the next step is clear: find a doctor willing to take these concerns seriously, conduct the scans, and let the evidence speak for itself.

But evidence alone can't capture what they've already taken—what they've already changed. The presence of an implant is proof of more than just their technology. It's proof of how far they've gone to invade my body, to tether me to their agenda, and to strip me of my privacy down to my cells. What began as night visits and strange dreams had now become something else entirely: a cold, persistent hand inside the sacred spaces of my biology.

There's a difference between being observed and being owned. Between being studied and being altered.

The implant may be hidden under my skin, but the real damage runs deeper. It reaches into the part of me that still wants to believe I'm free. It's in the anger that simmers beneath the surface—anger not just at them, but at the silence that surrounds all of this. At the world that keeps turning, unaware that some of us are being pulled apart, piece by piece.

That growing resentment would soon be matched by something far more painful—in those things about to be taken from me.

7

PIECES OF ME

The beginning of 2022 marked the start of a new relationship for me. Back in November 2020, I had taken my daughter Miranda to a local walk-in care clinic to satisfy some paperwork needed for her Medicaid-related health services and her in-home care provider, as managed by a social services agency with which I was working. During the appointment, Miranda's physician —whom I'll call Samantha—was having a conversation with me, during which I expressed my concerns about the COVID-19 and influenza vaccines the clinic was recommending. Given Miranda's complicated history with vaccine-related reactions, I shared the research I had gathered on these particular inoculations.

As we talked, I found myself unexpectedly taken by Samantha—by her calm, confident manner, her intelligence, and the warmth that came through despite the surgical mask covering half her face. Her tall, slender frame and captivating eyes stayed with me long after the appointment ended. There was something quietly magnetic about her. After we left the clinic, paperwork in hand, I remember wondering whether fate would allow me to cross paths with her again. It felt unlikely, but I couldn't help thinking about it.

Then, sometime about six months later in the summer of 2021, I received an email out of the blue—from Samantha. Apparently, several of her patients who had received the COVID vaccine were reacting horribly, including one case where a grand mal seizure was induced within minutes of the injection. She also noted a dramatic increase in what she referred to as "turbo cancers"—a spike so sudden and unexplainable that she questioned whether something larger was unfolding. She wanted to take me up on my previous offer to share any information I had gathered. I replied to her message, attaching several research documents and published medical articles I had archived.

She was grateful. Our exchange continued. We agreed to share anything new we came across in the future—and that simple agreement became the spark of something more. Over the next several months, our correspondence deepened. We began to talk regularly—first by email, then via text messages, and eventually through voice messages on WhatsApp. At the time, it was one of the more popular apps for smart phone users, and our conversations grew more personal with each passing week.

By January 2022, we had begun meeting in person for coffee and lunch dates during her days off. I found myself genuinely drawn to her—not just physically, but intellectually and emotionally. There was a depth to her I hadn't experienced in anyone else. I became smitten. And it was clear she felt the same way.

By February, we had become intimate. Neither of us had enjoyed the physical comfort of a loving relationship in quite some time. We were spending nights together at my house whenever we could, carving out a little island of joy in each other's company. We also spent time out in the world—exploring restaurants, taking walks in the park, and sharing one of her longtime passions: archery. She introduced me to it with enthusiasm, and it quickly became something we loved doing together. There was a lightness to those days, and a peace in simply being with her. I had never experienced a romance like it. We even had a shared nickname—Kindred—a fitting word for the connection we felt.

Sometime in late April, Samantha told me she had missed a

period and suspected she was pregnant. A home test confirmed it. The news came as a shock to both of us. I was 53 at the time, and she was in her early to mid-40s. While neither of us had planned for this, she told me she didn't believe in abortion. Considering how difficult it had been for her to conceive her two children years earlier—both through IVF—she felt perhaps this pregnancy was "meant to be." She would carry our child.

And I began, in my own quiet way, to come to terms with what that would mean. Emotionally. Practically. Spiritually. It wasn't the ideal time. I was older now—more tired than I used to be. But somewhere beneath the caution and anxiety, I felt a flicker of joy. I had always wanted more children. Life had interfered, and it often felt like that door had long since closed. But now, here was this chance—unexpected, maybe even miraculous.

I began picturing what life might look like with a new child. I imagined Miranda having a half-sibling. I imagined holding my baby in my arms again. And then just as quickly, I began worrying: Would I have the energy to raise a child at my age? Would I live long enough to see them graduate college? Could I afford to start over?

By late June, before she would have begun showing, Samantha miscarried. It happened in the ninth or tenth week. Despite my earlier excitement, I felt a surprising wave of relief. A part of me, the part tethered to practicality and time, felt that perhaps this was for the best. I had already given so much of myself to raising Miranda. Starting over would have demanded more than I felt I had left to give. Still, a quiet sadness settled in—a recognition that something had almost been, but now wasn't.

Samantha told me she had passed the tissues, but after careful inspection, she couldn't find the fetus or the fluid-filled sac. As a trained medical professional, she expected to find it. But it simply wasn't there. Confused, she consulted with her obstetrician and scheduled testing. I accompanied her to the second appointment, where the doctor confirmed she had indeed been pregnant—but that nothing remained inside her uterus. There were no complications. No retained tissue. She was healthy. That was our consolation.

Afterward, we processed the loss together. We both agreed that it was probably for the best. Her life was already stressful, and I was still recovering from years of nonstop caregiving. But despite how rational our decision sounded—despite how easily we both seemed to move on—I couldn't shake the feeling that something else had happened.

At the time, my "visitors" had still been active—showing up almost monthly. Their presence was unsettling, but routine in a strange way. And while I knew they had a persistent interest in reproductive material, I wasn't connecting them to what had happened with Samantha. I wondered, briefly, if the pregnancy might have drawn their attention somehow. But I didn't dwell on it. There was no evidence besides the missing fetus - only a vague unease. It remained just one more strange question in a life already filled with them.

In the end, I let it go. We both did. The missing fetus became a curiosity—a medical anomaly, unexplained but accepted. Life moved forward. And for a time, the subject faded into the background.

The Surgery

That very next month, in July of 2022 I was adjusting to life in the house without my daughter Miranda. She had just moved into a group home in Mundelein, Illinois in June with four other adult residents very much like her. I had the opportunity to tour the home and meet the other residents, including my daughter's new roommate named Morgan. Morgan was a young asian woman in her late 20's whose cognitive abilities and severity of autism matched my daughter's. But she had a very calm demeanor and was very curious of visitors to the home that I'd consider her 'friendly.' She would make a good roommate for Miranda and serve as a calming presence. This was important for me, as I was anxious about this move and wanted to see my daughter adjust well and be happy in her new home.

My house in July of 2022 was particularly quiet, save for my occasional AirBnB guest. I hadn't yet found employment after my daughter's departure, so I spent my spare time fixing up and cleaning the house. And for the first time ever, found that the house stayed clean without my daughter running about. In those days, my only real respite from the quiet was socializing with my best friend of the time, Angelo, who would visit Friday evenings to chat and have a drink, or I was spending time with my girlfriend Samantha.

On the night of Friday, July 15th, my friend Angelo had dropped by for our usual "kitchen party," where we put on some music, talk about whatever gossip he had in mind and sip a couple of cosmopolitans. "Cosmo's" were our drink at that time and usually after dispatching half a glass, we were laughing about something and forgetting our troubles. That night, however, Angelo couldn't stay late so it was decided he would depart about 10:30 p.m. and I chose to go to bed, having only had one drink. I wanted to get a good night's rest with the hopes that I could stain my back deck the following day. But it wasn't looking promising as Friday had been wet and raining.

By 11:00 p.m. I had gone to bed. My mind was a little restless at bedtime, obsessing over the details of my chore the next day. Had I purchased enough deck stain? Would it be too humid to power wash the deck and allow it to dry the same day? Did I remember all the needed supplies? These thoughts occupied my mind as it slowed, drowsiness clouding everything until sleep had dropped its veil, silencing all concerns.

There, in the blackness of my dreamless sleep, I became aware of pain in my left arm. My mind switched from blissful nothingness to pure awareness in a matter of seconds. Pain intruded my consciousness as my eyes opened. I was laying on my back and my arm was in such excruciating agony. My first instinct was to turn my head and look at my arm. And while I was able to move my head, I could move no other part of my body. I was paralyzed. What I saw next was horrific.

I was not in my bed. I was laying on a metal table in a dimly lit room, save for the brighter light that illuminated the table and the immediate area around it. As with other encounters, I could not discern a source for the lighting. Beyond the perimeter of this table was somewhat shadowed and grey. But that wasn't the horrific part.

Looking at my left arm, it was missing from just above the elbow! My arm was gone!

Alarmed and quite confused, and only able to move my head, I looked up and then to my right where I became aware of some individuals moving to the right of my table. But my eyes were having trouble focusing and they were beyond my lighted area, so I turned my head to the left and saw it. My arm, severed, was laying on a small metal cart next to my table. There was no blood! No blood coming out of my body and no blood surrounding my left arm on that cart. But I could see part of my humerus bone protruding an inch or so beyond the muscle tissues surrounding it. It reminded me of freshly butchered meat. But that was my meat! I was the one being butchered. How do I process this?!

The cart itself looked a little like stainless steel, but more pewter in color. It had a slightly raised, but smooth ridge at the perimeter as you'd expect on a coroner's table. The cart was approximately three feet long and perhaps 20 inches wide, on a single leg that brought it to the height of my table, which was perhaps three and a half to four feet off the floor.

As I experienced in previous encounters, my nervous system was squelched. Muted, if you prefer. If it hadn't been, I'm certain the pain would have been much worse as would have been my sense of panic. However, just as before, my fear response was almost nonexistent. I was naked and on a metal table, but I couldn't feel the cold metal on my skin. Was the metal cold? I'm accustomed to assuming that. Only my head and what was left of my arm had sensations. I wish that made sense.

I am reminded of my experience in the garage, where being in this state of sensory suspension prevented me from forming cogent thoughts. I had no words. Just a visual sense of awareness. And if my arm hadn't been severed, I doubt I would have felt a single thing. I doubt I would have awakened.

After noticing my arm on the cart and my shocked brain recording every visual detail as though my existence depended on it, I could hear someone approaching my table from the right. I lost consciousness just then, after having been awake for a mere 12 to 16 seconds. But those were the most impressionable seconds of my life. Have you ever been in a car accident where seconds before collision, time seemed to slow down and you were hyper focused on what you were seeing? To understand what my experience was like, you need only replicate that feeling, but remove eighty or ninety percent of your physical sensations, except for your sight.

I don't know what time I was taken from my house. When I awoke in my bed at home,

I looked at my arm to find it intact, but the elbow somewhat swollen. I searched for sutures or scars and found none. That doesn't seem possible. I sat up and looked at the clock across the room to see that it read 5:42 a.m. How long was I gone? I cradled my left elbow with my right palm. The elbow ached intensely. I had never had pain in a joint like this before. Testing my elbow, I was able to extend it about ninety percent. But not comfortably.

As I couldn't sleep any longer, I exited my room and showered, hoping the invigorating hot water would loosen me up a bit. However within an hour, my elbow had frozen completely at a ninety degree bend and the pain was too great to challenge that position. As the day progressed I experimented with both Tylenol and Advil so I could move about the house. But my hopes for staining the deck had been crushed for the time being.

Around noon that day, I called Angelo to tell him what happened. He picked up the phone using his usual greeting of "hello?" to which I replied "Hey, Ang, you're not going to believe what's happened!"

"What's going on Kiddo?" Angelo replied, using his favorite epithet for me, given our age difference.

"Ang, I was visited again last night. Except they took me this time." Angelo, familiar with my 'visits' at this point, was generally supportive as his own parents had an abduction experience in Cleveland, Ohio in their back yard in the 1960's. They saw a UFO in the sky, were approached from behind by something or someone, experienced hours of missing time and woke up in their patio chairs, each with multiple punctures on their arms, ribs and upper thighs.

"Why, what happened? Where was this? What did they do?" Angelo asked.

I spent the next five minutes describing the entire encounter as I have in the preceding paragraphs. I wanted to talk about it while the impressions were still fresh. I needed to talk about it. I was freaked out.

"I can't move my elbow, now." I added. "It's frozen stiff."

"Does it hurt?" he asked?

"Yeah, It aches, but it's tolerable as long as I don't try to move my elbow!" I answered.

"Are you going to get it looked at?" he asked.

"I probably will later, but what would I say? Aliens cut my frickin' arm off, give me some pain killers?" I suggested.

Angelo laughed, but suggested keeping that little detail to myself. "You should tell them you bumped it really hard. They'll look at it. You should get an X-Ray at least!"

I asked him if he would accompany me, but he was busy that weekend. The following day, I spoke with Samantha about what had happened. She was supportive and patient, as she had been throughout our relationship, and she seemed to believe me when I informed her about my visits. After listening quietly to my story, she asked, "Do you have any marks? Any scars?"

"No," I said, lifting the sleeve of my T-shirt and letting her examine my elbow. "Just swelling. No bruising. No cuts. Nothing."

She ran her fingers gently along the joint, pressing lightly. "It's definitely swollen," she said thoughtfully. "You should get an X-ray, just to be safe."

I nodded but said nothing. Samantha went on, her voice calm and clinical, "Since it happened overnight and there's no bruising, I don't think there's a break. Could be inflammation, or arthritis, or even a soft-tissue injury." She paused, looking up at me with concern. "If you want, you can schedule an appointment with my boss. He's your regular doctor anyway."

I appreciated her steadiness, her way of not making me feel crazy. But at the same time, there was an unspoken limit to how far she could follow me into this strange territory. And I had to respect that. She couldn't see what I had seen. She couldn't know what I knew. I thanked her, and she reassured me there was no immediate need for the emergency room. I considered her recommendation, but in the end, I chose not to pursue it.

Still, I never forgot the image of my severed arm on that metal cart—and how I could see the blunt white tip of my humerus bone exposed just above the elbow. It wasn't just the absence of blood that unsettled me. It was the way the bone protruded, clean and clinical, like the site of an extraction. Could they have taken bone marrow?

In the days that followed, still stunned by the lingering pain and the complete loss of motion in my elbow, I began researching what might cause such a reaction. I learned that while bone marrow is typically extracted from the iliac crest in the pelvis, emergency or experimental settings sometimes use the humerus instead.

The humerus is wrapped in vascular and nerve-rich tissue. Extracting marrow from it, especially near the midshaft or lower end, can trigger inflammation and pain that radiates directly into the elbow. I hadn't been injured in the conventional sense—no bruises, no cuts, no trauma I could point to. But if the Greys had drilled into the core of that bone while it was detached from my body—perhaps for genetic harvesting, or something else—I'd essentially suffered a procedure with no aftercare, no anesthesia, and no biological explanation I could give to a doctor. The more I read, the more it aligned. A deep, dull ache in the joint. Loss of range of motion. Localized swelling with no visible trauma. It was all there.

If they had removed marrow while my arm was severed, it would explain everything. And perhaps they knew it had caused more harm than intended. Because before the swelling had even begun to subside... they came back.

The Followup Visits

Over the next few days, I had to accustom myself to handling daily tasks using only my right arm. Everything from brushing my teeth to making coffee became a clumsy, one-handed performance. I found myself running errands and driving my red Chevy Trailblazer with just my right hand on the wheel. Thankfully, it was an automatic—I don't know how I would have managed with a stick shift. Even simple routines, like washing my hair in the shower, became exercises in awkward adaptation. Dispensing and applying shampoo with one hand felt almost ridiculous. I was forced to adjust, but everything reminded me that I wasn't whole. Something had changed.

A week passed. In the early hours of Saturday, July 23rd, I awoke to find myself in what I can only describe as a hospital-like setting. This time, I wasn't on a metal table but on a bed of some kind. It had a cushioned mattress covered in taut, white fabric that resembled soft canvas. There were no sheets or blankets—just the exposed, sterile bedding. I was lying on my back, head slightly propped up, and someone was holding my right hand.

At first, I thought I must be dreaming. My mind groped for logic, but nothing made sense. My left arm, surprisingly, was fully extended out to my left. I could feel it—but I couldn't move it. Nor could I move anything else, except for a little motion in my right hand and arm. I turned to see who was beside me, holding my hand.

What I saw didn't match who I was expecting.

At first glance, it looked like a girl or a young woman—small in stature, with delicate hands and bare feet that only reached to my calves. But as my eyes moved up toward her face, I realized what I was actually looking at. This wasn't a human. It was a small grey.

She gazed at me calmly, her large, dark eyes locking with mine. Then, without moving her lips, I heard her voice inside my mind: "Do you have something you want to tell me?"

I didn't. I was so confused—why was she holding my hand? What did she mean by that question? What did she expect me to say? My thoughts swirled, but I couldn't form a reply. I simply stared back at her in silence, trying to understand what was happening. Then I felt it—two hands taking hold of my left arm at the elbow and forearm.

Turning my head to the left, I saw another figure—this one towering, easily over seven feet tall. A tall grey, much larger than Syczilick, leaned over the left side of the bed, inspecting my arm with quiet focus. Its hands moved with clinical precision, carefully manipulating the elbow joint and studying its range of motion.

I was about to turn back toward the girl to ask what they were doing—why they were here—when I lost consciousness. The moment vanished like vapor.

I woke later that morning, much later than I usually do after an encounter. The sun had already risen, casting pale light into my room. The clock read 5:45 a.m. My elbow still ached and was visibly swollen, but I noticed something had shifted. I could now move it slightly—maybe ten degrees in either direction from the fixed right-angle bend where it had been stuck. It wasn't much, but it was progress. Sitting up in bed, feet dangling just above the floor, I stared downward, trying to make sense of it all.

What was that all about? Who was the girl? Were they checking up on my arm? And what did she want me to tell her?

As the fog lifted and my thoughts became clearer, I kept circling back to one conclusion: whatever they had done when they severed my arm, it had left some kind of damage—damage they felt compelled to monitor, or maybe even repair. Was that tall grey performing some kind of corrective procedure? Was this encounter their version of a follow-up visit?

That suspicion only grew stronger a week later, when it happened again. Three visits in three weeks!

This time, I awoke in a standing position, naked, facing a grey wall lined with a pewter-colored railing. It reminded me of the kind you'd see along the wall of a dance studio. My legs were weak but functional. A tall grey stood beside me, gently guiding me by the shoulder toward the railing. I instinctively knew what was expected of me: to place my hands on the rail and steady myself.

Even in my foggy, half-conscious state, I recognized the rhythm of it—this was a routine. A system. I obeyed, still unable to speak, still unable to form more than fragmented thoughts.

The tall grey now stood to my right. Without a word, it turned me gently to face it, then reached out with both hands and began inspecting my left arm again. Just like the week before, its fingers glided along the length of my forearm and elbow, repeating the motion several times. I could feel pressure, but it didn't hurt. Its hands moved deliberately, like a physical therapist testing the stability of a joint.

In that moment, I felt like a dementia patient. I could see. I could move when directed. But I couldn't speak. I had so many questions. So many things I wanted to say. But whatever control they exerted over me, it suppressed my expressive thought—just like it had during the garage encounter two years earlier.

It wasn't just my arm they had taken. It was access to myself. My ability to communicate, to resist, to comprehend what was happening. Whatever force they used to entrance me... it didn't just paralyze the body—it muted the will.

They were not interested in what I had to say. They never were.

I had adapted to the pain. I had adjusted to the silence. But what lingered most wasn't just what they'd done to my body—it was what they kept from me. My voice. My will. My right to understand. Whatever they were doing to me, it wasn't finished. And somewhere deep inside, I had begun to sense that this wasn't just a sequence of isolated events. It was a dismantling—quiet, methodical, and personal. Something was being taken from me... one piece at a time.

Other Reports of Alien Surgery

As disturbing as my experiences were, I've since come to understand they are not entirely unique. Other abductees have reported procedures that mirror aspects of what happened to me—accounts that span decades, continents, and demographics. These stories, like mine, describe not only medical intervention, but something colder and more calculated: the harvesting of parts, the intrusion into the most sacred chambers of the body, and the unsettling silence that always follows.

Whitley Strieber, in *Transformation* and *The Secret School*, recounted his own experiences of being operated on while immobilized. In one of his more vivid memories, he described a needle inserted into his brain through the roof of his mouth—a procedure that left no external trace but carried a weight of trauma he couldn't shake. In another, he was restrained while something sharp was inserted behind his eye. He too described the same eerie suppression of fear and pain, replaced with an observational stillness that left him unable to resist or even cry out.

Then there are the tissue extractions reported by numerous abductees investigated by Budd Hopkins and Dr. David Jacobs. One of the most common physical aftermaths are scoop marks—small, cleanly removed patches of flesh, usually from the leg or arm. These indentations often appear overnight and are noted for their surgical precision. Jacobs speculated that they may involve the removal of skin samples, nerve tissue, or even DNA-laden fluid. No pain. No bleeding. Just a piece of the person—gone.

In *The Threat* and *Walking Among Us,* Jacobs discusses cases where abductees were subjected to gynecological procedures or sperm extraction while under control, often in conditions eerily similar to mine. Many of these individuals describe an environment that resembles a sterile clinic, with beds or tables that feel more like platforms than furniture, and lighting that seems to emanate from nowhere. The procedures are described as emotionless, clinical, and completely one-sided. And like me, they wake in their homes with no visible signs of surgery—just pain, swelling, stiffness, or the afterglow of something they can't explain.

Even more chilling are the accounts collected by Linda Moulton Howe, who drew parallels between human abduction surgeries and the patterns found in cattle mutilations—where soft tissue is removed with laser-like precision, often from the jaw, eye, genitals, and rectum, and always without a drop of blood. The implication is hard to ignore: the same beings conducting silent harvests on animals may also be collecting from us.

Some experiencers have reported visible marks, implants, or even incisions that vanish within days. Others, like myself, are left with joint stiffness or deep tissue pain that lingers for weeks. But most disturbing of all is what we're not left with—answers.

These procedures are not framed as medical care. They are not for our benefit. They are acts of collection. Of manipulation. And in nearly all of these stories, something is taken. Whether it's bone marrow, sperm, eggs, flesh, or something less tangible, the pattern is consistent.

We lose a piece of ourselves—quietly, efficiently, without consent. When I reflect on what was done to my arm, and the strange disappearance of the child Samantha and I briefly expected, I realize that my story doesn't stand alone. It's part of a larger pattern—one that spans the globe, hidden in plain sight. And it raises a chilling possibility: what if these aren't just experiments? What if these procedures are steps in a long, deliberate process we're only beginning to understand?

8

PIECES LEFT BEHIND

Some time at the end of the first week of September, on the 7th or 8th, I remember waking up in a standing position inside a room with pewter-colored walls, accompanied by two tall Greys. As per usual in these encounters, I was disoriented and mentally fogged—a state I've come to recognize as a deliberate suppression of conscious thought during these experiences. My ability to react emotionally or critically analyze what was happening felt muted, as if I were intoxicated.

Before me was a featureless wall, smooth and metallic, with no visible seams or screens. One of the Greys directed my attention toward it, indicating that I was about to see something important. I was asked to look at the wall so I could see what my offspring looked like. The phrasing struck me as oddly clinical, and yet, in the moment, I simply obeyed.

As soon as I fixed my gaze to the blank surface, three rows of rectangular images appeared, displaying faces of varying ages. The display reminded me of a digital screen, yet there were no borders, no flickering pixels, no indication that any technology had produced it. It was as if the wall itself had transformed into a window, showing me something beyond its surface. The images weren't flat, like a typical photograph. They had depth, like a hologram, and the longer I looked, the more I felt that these faces were not mere projections.

They were real.

Despite the clarity of the images at the time, I find that now, I cannot recall their facial details. What I do remember is their varying ages—some appearing as toddlers, others as teenagers, and at least a few as fully grown adults. The implications were staggering. Whatever has been happening to me, it would appear that it has been occurring for far longer than I had previously realized.

At that moment, I turned to my escorts and asked, *"What are their names? Do they have names?"*

One of the Greys responded with a question of its own: *"Would you like to give them names?"*

The question caught me off guard, but in my mentally dulled state, I took it at face value. I said, *"Sure."* But rather than carefully considering meaningful names, my mind defaulted to what was most accessible and familiar—characters from the original series of Star Trek.

"Let's call this one Kirk, and this one Spock, and this one McCoy."

In rapid succession, I rattled off every ridiculous name I could think of, assigning them to the faces with the flippancy of someone trying to amuse themselves in an absurd situation. If I had been in my right mind, I might have chosen dignified names—something timeless, something meaningful. But in that moment, none of this felt real to me, even as I stood there, naming my supposed offspring.

The Greys, however, seemed amused. I could sense their awareness that I was referencing popular human culture. There was no chastisement or disapproval, only a vague sense of detached curiosity, as if they found my reaction interesting in some abstract way.

Still, something tells me these children of mine never learned of the names I randomly assigned to them.

Other Abductees & the Hybrid Presentation

Later, when I awoke in my bed, the weight of the experience hit me in full. I had been given an opportunity to understand my involvement, to see the faces of those I helped create—and yet, in the moment, I had treated it like a joke. Why?

This wasn't the first time abductees had reported being shown their hybrid offspring, nor would it be the last. Budd Hopkins, David Jacobs, and Whitley Strieber all documented similar cases—men and women brought aboard ships, led to nursery-like environments or shown images of hybrid children, often with disturbing emotional detachment in the moment, only to be struck by the enormity of it later.

In Budd Hopkins' research, abductees—particularly women—reported being presented with their hybrid children and asked to interact with them in some way. Some were encouraged to hold and comfort the children, while others were simply shown their faces on a screen-like display, much like what I experienced. David Jacobs documented a pattern in which abductees were repeatedly introduced to the same hybrid children over multiple encounters, as if the Greys were testing human parental instincts or reinforcing a psychological connection.

Whitley Strieber described a moment in which he was presented with small, frail-looking children who seemed partially human but unmistakably different. He was given no explanation, only the implication that they were connected to him. Meanwhile, Dolores Cannon, through hypnotic regression, uncovered accounts of abductees witnessing souls being inserted into hybrid bodies—as if the Greys were not only engineering new beings biologically but also spiritually.

The consistency of these reports made my own experience even more unnerving. Were the Greys presenting these children to me for a reason, or was this merely a psychological experiment—observing how I would react?

A Moment Lost in the Fog

Unlike the mothers described in Hopkins' and Jacobs' research, I felt no natural parental bond toward these beings in the moment. I did not feel joy, sorrow, or love. It was only after I awoke in my bed that I began to process what had truly happened. Why had I not reacted more seriously? Why did the emotional gravity only strike me after the fact?

This emotional detachment appears to be a consistent aspect of abduction experiences, almost as if the Greys intentionally suppress natural human reactions. It makes me wonder: Are they incapable of understanding human parental instincts? Are they attempting to learn how to cultivate emotions in hybrids? Or are they simply manipulating our psychology, keeping us in a trance-like state so we don't react with panic or resistance? I cannot shake the feeling that, had I been fully awake, I would have reacted very differently. Perhaps that is why they never allow us to be fully awake. And why they come to us from the shadows.

The Questions That Haunt Me

Later that morning, as I sat up in bed, I tried desperately to recall their faces—but the details were already slipping from me. It was as if their images had been erased, leaving behind only the knowledge that I had seen them.

I had been shown something profoundly important, yet I had been kept in a state where I could not fully absorb or react to it. And then, the bigger questions emerged. What is their purpose? Why are they being bred? Where do they call home? These are not idle curiosities—they are questions that burn inside me, demanding answers that never seem to come.

But one thing is certain: they are out there, my children - and they exist.

May 2022 and October 2022: My Chats with Linda Moulton Howe

By May of 2022, during the height of my recurring encounters, I was feeling increasingly isolated and in need of guidance. I had spoken to a few people by then—people I trusted or thought might be open—but there's a difference between venting and finding someone who truly understands. I needed someone who had heard stories like mine before, who could tell me whether I was losing my grip or brushing up against something real.

During this time, I had fallen into a kind of research frenzy. I was devouring documentaries on Amazon Prime, streaming programs on Netflix, and binge-watching Ancient Aliens—not out of idle curiosity, but as a lifeline. I wasn't trying to entertain myself. I was searching for validation. For clues. For language to wrap around the impossible.

Among the experts featured, one person stood out. Time and again, she spoke with clarity, seriousness, and a depth of knowledge that went far beyond the usual soundbites. That person was Linda Moulton Howe.

A former investigative reporter, Linda gained national attention in the 1980s with her groundbreaking documentary A Strange Harvest, which explored the mystery of cattle mutilations with journalistic integrity and courage. Her work, which earned her a regional Emmy, was a rare example of someone bringing legitimate investigative chops to a field too often dismissed as fringe. Over the decades, she's reported on whistleblowers from within the military-industrial complex, alien technology, abduction cases, government secrecy, and the broader mystery of non-human intelligence. Through her long-running website, *Earthfiles*, she has become a central figure in the world of high-integrity UFO research.

So I did something I wasn't sure would go anywhere: I went to Earthfiles.com, found her contact information, and sent her a thoughtful email explaining who I was and what I'd experienced. To my surprise, she wrote back.

Her tone was warm, professional, and genuinely curious. Within a week, we had scheduled a phone call. I remember pacing my home that day, both nervous and relieved—like I was finally about to speak with someone who might be able to make sense of all this.

That first call lasted two hours. Linda listened carefully as I laid out the core of my experiences. While nothing I shared was new to me by that point, there was one moment in our conversation that struck me with its immediacy.

When I told her about the orbs from my childhood—how they entered through my closet door and seemed to interact with me directly—she responded with a calm but firm statement that stayed with me.

"Erik," she said, "as soon as you mentioned how the orbs came through your closet door, I knew you were telling the truth. That one little detail aligns so well with other abductees I've interviewed who've told me the exact same thing. And these aren't details that are widely publicized. That's how I know you're sincere."

Hearing those words, from someone of Linda's stature, meant more to me than I could say in the moment. She wasn't humoring me. She wasn't offering empty validation. She was saying, "I've heard this before. You're not alone."

It gave me the courage to speak more openly. It gave me the momentum to keep going.

Five months later, in October of 2022, Linda reached out to me again—this time, with a specific question. She asked if we could schedule another call, and of course, I agreed.

During that second conversation, which also stretched to nearly two hours, Linda asked me directly: "Have you ever been shown apocalyptic imagery? Have the Greys ever given you visions of catastrophic events?"

I paused and searched my memory. The answer was no. At least, not that I could remember. What I did recall, however, was a peculiar moment from an encounter I had left out of previous chapters. In this incident, I was walking alongside a tall Grey, following the wall of a corridor, positioned on the inside of the path. We were moving quietly when the being said, "You need to get rid of your nuclear weapons."

My response, baffling in retrospect, was: "If we do that, we give up our mutual deterrent! We can't do that."

When I woke from that encounter, I was stunned—not by the content of the interaction, but by my own reply. I don't believe in nuclear weapons. I don't believe they are necessary as a deterrent. I believe they're the kind of bluff no one should ever call, a catastrophic trump card with no winner. So why did I respond that way? Where did that come from?

I now suspect that I wasn't speaking from my higher mind—but from a fogged, manipulated state. One where I wasn't thinking clearly. And that's one of the reasons I resent these beings so deeply. I never get to be the full version of myself with them. My mind is constantly fogged, my cognition filtered through their control. I think that's why they see me as uncooperative. Because I am. Because I hate being manipulated.

I shared this story with Linda, explaining that it was the closest thing I had to the "apocalyptic vision" theme she had asked about. She listened closely and agreed it might point to deeper programming—or maybe something I've yet to fully recover.

Whatever the case, I was glad we spoke again. Linda is an engaging conversationalist—thoughtful, wise, and generous with her insights. Talking with her feels like speaking to someone who's been walking the same road, just a little farther ahead. It helped to know she was curious enough to follow up, to ask more, to want to understand.

It also gave me insight into something I'd later hear from a producer at Ancient Aliens who had worked with her many times: "There's no such thing as a short conversation with Linda." If my experience is any proof, that's true. And honestly? That's not a bad thing at all.

June 2023: The Baby Presentation

In the months following my encounter where the Greys had shown me images of my many hybridized offspring, I had experienced a few significant life changes. In November of 2022, I managed to secure full-time employment as a graphic designer at a national product distribution company near O'Hare Airport. This was a much-needed change, as I had been an empty nester for six months and was no longer receiving my daughter's social security income, which had previously helped me cover my bills. Financially, things had become challenging, but with this job, I was finally finding stability again.

Then, in January of 2023, Samantha and I parted ways in a breakup that was entirely against my wishes. I was genuinely in love with her, but circumstances never worked in our favor. Our relationship had been strained by factors neither of us could fully control, and though I tried to hold on, the separation became inevitable. The loss lingered like a dull ache beneath the surface of my daily life, but by mid-year, I had at least managed to regain some footing. A few months later, I was able to finance a new automobile, and with my job keeping me busy, I felt like I was getting back on my feet—situationally, financially, and at least on the surface, emotionally.

Then, in early June of 2023, I was abducted again. Or, as I like to say, I was taken on another involuntary field trip.

I became conscious in a standing position aboard what I assume was a spacecraft. My awareness returned not with the sluggish confusion of a dream, but with an eerie suddenness, as though a light switch had flipped in my mind. Before me stood a tall Grey, its large black eyes studying me in silence. The room around me was circular, expansive, with a diameter of what I estimate to be fifty or sixty feet. Encircling the room were wide, horizontally stretched windows that were vertically narrow, creating a panoramic band around the space. The outside was dark, an emptiness beyond the glass that gave no indication of where we were—or how high above the Earth, if at all.

In my entranced state, my mind struggled to rationalize the environment, attempting to make sense of what I was seeing. I wasn't in a spacecraft, I thought. I was in an air traffic control tower. And the tall Grey before me—it wasn't an alien. It was just a very tall man. This distortion of perception is something I've experienced before, an artificial overlay of logic that seems meant to calm the abductee or obscure the reality of the situation.

But whatever illusion was at play, it could not hide the focal point of the room.

At its center, resting atop a smooth metallic table, was a baby.

The child, no more than six or seven months old, was facing away from me, making it impossible to see his face. Even so, I could tell from his size and posture that he was a boy. He was actively moving, shifting between sitting and crawling, his tiny hands exploring the surface of the table with the innocent curiosity of an infant.

Then the Grey spoke, its words ringing clearly inside my head—not spoken aloud, but delivered directly into my mind with the unmistakable precision of telepathic communication.

"He's yours," it said.

The words struck me with a strange detachment. I understood what it meant, but my emotions remained muted, as though the full significance of the statement had not yet reached me.

The Grey continued. "But he has a genetic problem, and you're here to provide the tissues we need to correct it."

"A genetic problem." The phrase lingered in my thoughts, igniting a flicker of confusion beneath the surface of my trance. The Grey's tone carried no alarm, no concern—just a simple, matter-of-fact statement. But the words bothered me, even as my mind struggled to form questions.

Genetic problem? What does that mean? I wanted to ask. I needed to know. But before I could, my consciousness was abruptly cut off.

One moment I was standing in the room, staring at the baby on the table. The next, I was gone. Switched off like some kind of machine.

The Awakening & The Realization

I awoke to the shrill chime of my alarm, my body rigid and my mind heavy with exhaustion. The clock read 5:30 a.m., signaling the start of another day. But as I sat up in bed, something felt off.

My body ached, not from physical strain, but from an indescribable fatigue, as though I had not slept at all. My limbs were leaden, my head clouded, and the faint echoes of the encounter still swirled in my mind, as vivid as a memory yet distant, as if I had experienced it in another lifetime.

And then, as the weight of the experience began to settle, the sadness hit me. I had been shown my own child—my son—and I wasn't even allowed to hold him.

The realization stung in a way that bypassed logic and struck directly at the heart. He was mine, and yet, he was not mine at all. A child I had helped create, a child who should have been with me, was instead lying on a table in the custody of beings who had taken him from me before I had even known of his existence.

And then another thought struck me—a thought so chilling, so sudden, it was as if a cold wind had swept through my mind. The baby was six or seven months old. I did the math.

The previous year, when Samantha had miscarried our baby, she had told me that it would have been born around my birthday in January of 2023. That was six months ago. My heart sank. "Oh, God." Could this baby have been Samantha's as well? The timing fit too perfectly.

The Greys take the fetus in its ninth or tenth week, gestate it artificially to full-term, and he's "born" in January—just not through Samantha's birth canal. Then, six months later, they show him to me. A storm of emotions overtook me. The woman I had loved—the woman I still loved—might be the mother of this child. We had a baby together. And yet, we didn't. He was taken from us.

My thoughts raced with questions that had no answers. What had they done to him? Had they altered him? Had they hybridized him during gestation, manipulating his DNA for their own purposes? And was this the reason for his so-called genetic problem?

I wish I were telling you this as a lead-in to a later revelation, a moment where I would eventually learn the answers. But I cannot. To this day, those answers elude me. And with them, so does the child I was never allowed to know.

I would have given him a beautiful name.

Reflecting on the subtexts

As I sat at my desk later that morning, trying to focus on my work, my thoughts kept circling back to the experience. The child was real. Flesh and blood. I had seen him move, seen him exploring the surface of the table like any ordinary baby might. But the way in which I had been shown him—suddenly, without warning, without context—felt deliberate. Like a test.

And then, a realization hit me. The Children on the Wall!

Months earlier, the Greys had shown me images of my hybridized offspring, projected onto a seamless metallic wall as if they were nothing more than portraits in a gallery. At the time, my reaction had been flippant, my mind fogged and disconnected. I had rattled off names from Star Trek without any sense of the gravity of what I was being shown. The Greys had watched me do it.

Could they have perceived my lack of attachment? Could they have realized that static images were not enough to make me process the weight of what was happening? And if so... could this encounter —the presentation of my living, breathing son—have been their next attempt?

This time, there were no screens, no detached images. Instead, they placed me in a room with him. They let me see him move, hear the soft rustling of his limbs, watch the way he interacted with his environment.

Had this been their way of testing my reaction? To see if a living child would break through my fogged perception in a way that holographic images had not?

If so... what did they learn? The answer, perhaps, is that they still controlled the outcome.

I had not been allowed to touch him. I had not even been allowed to see his face. The moment I might have stepped closer, the moment

I might have reached out—they had ended the encounter. They did not want to risk a response they could not predict. They were observing something—but what?

Was it my emotional connection to him? My genetic compatibility? Were they trying to determine whether their hybrid offspring could trigger the same bonding instincts as a human child? Or were they simply trying to see if I would react at all? The worst part is that I don't know. I may never know.

In the days that followed, the questions wouldn't let go. If they're showing me my children—then where are they being raised? Where do they live, play, grow? These aren't phantom images—they are physical, developing beings. And if they're not being nurtured by human parents, then by whom? But it's not just the mystery that haunts me. It's the loss.

It took me a long time to name the feeling. At first, I told myself I wasn't angry. I wasn't grieving. I just felt... hollowed out. Like something deeply meaningful had been drained from my life before I'd even known to reach for it. But the more I let myself sit with it—truly feel it—the more I understood what was really there.

I feel cheated.

Not just in the biological sense. Not just because my genetic material was taken. But because I'm not just a sperm donor—I'm a father. A good one. I raised a daughter with care, with sacrifice, with devotion that cut me to the bone and still left room for more. I knew what fatherhood meant. And I wanted more children. I had it in me to love them. To guide them. To witness them become.

Instead, I was kept at a distance from the very experience of fatherhood they now claimed I had fulfilled. I wasn't absent—I was raising a child with every ounce of my being. But I still had more to give. I had the heart, the patience, the strength to love more children, to raise them, guide them, protect them. And instead of that life unfolding naturally, I was shown the outcome of something stolen—offspring I would never hold, never name, never love in any human way. Children who exist, perhaps, in physical health and engineered design—but without the sacred thread that connects a parent to a child. Without bedtime stories or scraped knees or whispered encouragements through tears. Without me.

That's what stings the most. That I was deemed useful, but not necessary. That they took what they needed and gave nothing in return—not even the dignity of seeing me as more than a lab rat.

And yes, when I let it settle, I do grieve. I grieve for the children who will never know they were wanted in a way the Greys could never fabricate. I grieve for the life I might have had—filled with laughter, mess, complexity, and warmth—and for the legacy that now lives apart from me, silent and unreachable. And I am angry. Not the kind of anger that explodes. The kind that settles in the bones like cold iron. The kind that says: I deserved better than this.

They showed me what was taken from me as if it were an act of closure. But it wasn't closure—it was a wound left open. A reminder that they never saw me as a father, only as a resource. And no matter how many sterile hallways they walk me down, no matter how many children they manufacture with my name in their genetic code, they will never know what they truly stole. The unsettling possibility crept into my thoughts with growing persistence: these hybrids may not be somewhere far away. They may be here—beneath us—already waiting.

9

BENEATH US, OUR FUTURE

The summer of 2023 was a dizzying time in my life, as it seemed my visitors were not slowing down their visits, keeping to their general four to six week schedule. July would be no different, as it turned out. Just the month before, I was shown a child that likely belonged to both Samantha and me and I was struggling with the emotions and implications of that revelation. I also struggled with whether to tell Samantha, not that doing so would serve any benefit. While she was receptive to the fact of my 'visitations,' and believed my accountings of each incident, I feared that if I told her about our son, she might receive the news with skepticism, possibly as some ploy to speak with her as a means of restarting our relationship. As a result, my hesitation persisted and I never spoke of it.

In the latter half of July, I was taken from my bed once again and became semi-conscious in a sitting position in a room very much like the one where I had been shown a wall containing images of my offspring, the previous year. And much like that encounter, I recall being in the presence of two tall greys. My confusion during this encounter was pronounced. I cannot remember the premise for my being there, or the specifics of my exchanges with the two greys. All I can recall is a portion of a conversation. I remember that I asked about my offspring, as the memory of meeting my son was fresh in my mind. I remember asking why I couldn't be with my children, and that I was upset with them. The response I received was somewhat derogatory. I was told my children were only "half hairy ape," and that they couldn't live in my society. I didn't understand why they would say something like that, but I surmise that they were annoyed with me. Perhaps before my memory of that incident began, when I became conscious enough, I had been rude or mean toward them?

I accepted their explanation relating why my children couldn't join me, but I wanted to know more. I asked the two greys where, exactly, my children were being kept. At that moment, I was invited to stand and was motioned toward a grey, smooth wall - much like the one where I was shown my numerous offspring the year before. On the wall, a 3-dimensional map appeared. I recognized it immediately. It was a map of the 48 contiguous united states! And it featured all the state division lines. That was unexpected.

The image of the map enlarged as though to zoom in on Illinois and its surrounding region, but at a 45 degree angle. I could see Lake Michigan, the bottom portions of Wisconsin and Michigan... I could see the eastern parts of Iowa and Missouri and western Indiana. And within Illinois, appeared what I perceived as large, constructed subterranean caverns, running parallel with each other, from north to south just west of the Indiana border.

There were three caverns. Two running parallel at the same depth, perhaps one third to half a mile below the surface, and one slightly deeper, situated between them. They were all fatter in their centers, and tapered at their ends, with their southern ends all sloping downward. My first thought was to compare their shapes to three bananas, though flatter in their curvature. These caverns, as depicted, were HUGE. At the north end, they began just a little bit south of Chicago's South Side... about even with the bottom of Lake Michigan and came as far south as Peoria, Illinois. Such caverns could host a lot of people. Enough to fill a city, easily.

I lost consciousness shortly after seeing the map. I got to examine it for seven to ten seconds, I can't remember precisely how long. But it's etched into my memory and I can still see it.

Upon waking back at home, I sat up in my bed with the map fresh in my mind. While it was strangely comforting to learn that my offspring were nearby and not on some other strange world, the revelation created more questions than it answered. For instance, how are such caverns possible? If these exist, how are they unknown? The only caverns I'm aware of are close to St. Louis. How can anyone possibly remove and displace so much material without being detected? Caverns that large must have displaced enough rock to rival the panama canal. But more profound than the technical aspects of these caverns, if they exist, is the implications raised by their existence.

I take it as fact that the greys are breeding a hybrid race of people. "Half hairy ape," as they chided and half something else. However, the existence of these caverns - and the reason they were shown to me - would suggest that these hybrids are being kept locally. And if that is the case, does that mean that they're being bred to LIVE on the Earth? I've since read speculations in my research where others proposed that human-grey hybrids were being created to save their own species that had lost the ability to procreate sexually. The assumption, being, that they'd take their new offspring to their own world. But these caverns would suggest otherwise. The sheer size of those caverns suggest to me that they are basing their breeding operations in subterranean installations like these, possibly around the globe. I might speculate that it makes sense to base operations near large population centers, such as Chicago. They would be closer to their breeding stock! But then again, with their technology, distance is hardly an obstacle. Perhaps the location of these caverns are based upon the type of rock that exists in Illinois bedrock? And the fact that this region is geologically very stable, given that earthquakes are rare?

Confronted with these questions, I decided to take a closer look at the feasibility of such caverns in the location I was shown. If I can't prove they exist, maybe I can learn whether they're at least POSSIBLE. If an analysis shows it is possible, or if there are any advantages to the design and placement as I was shown, then perhaps the map was real and not something I could dream up. If these caverns were smartly designed, that could add gravitas to the memory.

Geological Feasibility of the Caverns

The first thing I considered was the bedrock composition of eastern Illinois, particularly west of the Indiana border, where the caverns appeared to be located. What I found was interesting. The dominant bedrock in that region is dolostone, a sedimentary carbonate rock similar to limestone but with a higher magnesium content. It forms in marine environments and is known for being structurally strong and resistant to erosion, meaning it could theoretically support large underground chambers. Unlike looser, more porous rock, dolostone wouldn't just collapse under its own weight if enormous caverns had been carved into it.

Dolostone has long been quarried and mined, and large underground voids have already been created in similar rock formations. There are limestone and dolostone mines across the Midwest, and many have been repurposed for storage facilities, military operations, and even underground cities. The stability of this rock—paired with the fact that Illinois isn't prone to major earthquakes—makes it an ideal candidate for subterranean construction.

Considering the design of the caverns, it was too deliberate, too structured to be anything but engineered. Three vast chambers, running parallel beneath Illinois, weren't something that nature could have carved out on its own. Their layout suggests a specific function.

The two upper caverns sat at the same depth, stretching north to south, widest at their centers, and tapering at the ends. Below them, a third cavern lay positioned between the two but deeper underground. All three sloped downward at their southern ends, which struck me as an important detail. The more I examined it, the more I realized how much purpose may be embedded in that design.

The parallel structure of the upper two caverns would ensure even weight distribution, reducing the risk of collapse. The third, deeper cavern between them could serve a structural buffer role, preventing stress fractures or pressure buildup. Or maybe it was something else entirely—an underground transport route, a storage facility, or a way to move between the upper chambers without disrupting whatever was happening inside them.

And then there was the slope. The downward tilt at the southern ends of all three caverns couldn't be a coincidence. Water is always an issue underground, and in an operation of this scale, drainage would be a necessity. If water collected anywhere, it would naturally flow southward, away from critical areas. Maybe they had reservoirs, a controlled runoff system, or even ways to repurpose the water for their needs. I also found another possibility—airflow. In enclosed spaces, heavier gases like carbon dioxide tend to settle. A sloped design could have been a way to direct air circulation, keeping the environment controlled and breathable.

And what about the depth? I looked at that as well. While I cannot be certain what the depth was by just a glance at the map, I would estimate it was about one third of a mile deep, possibly half a mile, maximum. Somewhere between 1,700 and 2,500 feet. Interestingly, in recent months, I went a step further. I examined geological surveys of Eastern Illinois—specifically the region west of the Indiana border where I remembered seeing the caverns. What I found only deepened my conviction. At depths of 1,700 to 2,600 feet, the underlying bedrock in that corridor is composed of Mississippian and Devonian carbonates—primarily dolostone and limestone—both of which are structurally competent and historically known to host deep solutional voids. According to the Illinois State Geological Survey and associated U.S. Geological Survey data, there is nothing in the published geological record that precludes the existence of caverns at those depths. In fact, such carbonate formations—lying below hundreds of feet of glacial overburden—could feasibly harbor large hollowed spaces without detection. These formations are the same types used for oil and gas storage, military bunkers, and even deep CO_2 sequestration sites. And due to the limited resolution of deep seismic surveys in rural areas, such voids, even if massive, could remain invisible to all but the most targeted geological investigations.

While I can't be certain of the exact alignment, based on my memory of the map, the caverns seemed to begin roughly at the latitude of the south end of Lake Michigan and extended southward, perhaps as far as Bloomington. If that's accurate, they would span a corridor beneath counties such as **Will, Kankakee, Grundy, Livingston, Iroquois, Ford, Champaign, and Vermilion**, forming a north–south band just west of the Indiana border. It's a region not known for natural caverns—there are no documented karst zones there—but that's precisely what made the revelation so strange and so fascinating. I may never be able to prove the existence of those caverns, but the geological evidence clearly shows that their existence isn't fantasy—it's plausible. And if it's plausible, then what I was shown might not have been metaphor or manipulation. It might have been real.

What's more, the counties that overlay the corridor I described—Will, Iroquois, Vermilion, Douglas, Coles, and Cumberland—sit outside Illinois' traditional oil belt. The majority of the state's petroleum drilling has historically occurred much farther south, in counties like Marion, White, and Crawford. This means the region beneath eastern Illinois has seen relatively little deep borehole exploration. With fewer well logs and less incentive for high-resolution seismic surveys, the chances of detecting large underground anomalies—like the caverns I was shown—would be slim. If anything, the lack of oil activity in this part of the state leaves a vast blind spot beneath the surface. And that blind spot might just be hiding something.

What would the ambient temperature be at that depth, I wondered? Doing some research, I learned about something called the "geothermal gradient," which adds heat the deeper you go below the surface. If we start with the average surface temperature for Eastern Illinois, which is about 50-54 degrees, Fahrenheit, and add heat as we go underground, the gradient adds 25 to 30 degrees celcius per kilometer. Between a third of a mile and half a mile, you're looking at ambient temperatures anywhere from 75 to 95 degrees, Fahrenheit. Year round. If I'm wrong about the depth, and it was shallower, the temperatures could be more comfortable for human habitation. Any deeper than a third of a mile would require active cooling for human habitation.

All of these geological and design considerations, while still speculative, would suggest that there is more to this map than what my imagination could present in a dream scenario. Why do I even bring that up? While I remember being awake in a semi-conscious state and am fully content to accept it was a genuine encounter like the others, I gave it additional scrutiny because it's something that can be investigated. A tangible, physical detail that could be proven or disproven. The map gave me a location and a design. While I don't have seismic equipment to try to detect voids a third of a mile into the bedrock... and I certainly don't have any ability to access these caverns (assuming their existence), there is at least the possibility for analyzing what I was shown, more closely. Since I am not a geologist, my cursory examination detailed here satisfies me for the time being. However, I welcome commentary should an expert read these pages. And if anyone wants to hunt for evidence beneath our feet, I'd be fascinated. I say this, fully understanding that if the existence of these caverns were disproven, it could throw my credibility right down a well. But then, so many of the things I'm reporting to you in this book are a tough sell to science-minded skeptics.

A History, Below

As I've been exploring every aspect of my abduction encounters, seeking out modern and historical precedence - eager to understand what's happened to me and why, I decided to use my memoir as a means of investigation. To not only share my memories, but to discuss what I have learned in my journey of discovery.

While it interests me to know the purpose for being shown a map of these caverns - the location of my genetic offspring and a local base of operations for a breeding program - it occurred to me that I've heard many examples within UFOlogy and ancient alien theory where people had reported subterranean bases used by aliens, or those assumed to be gods.

My experience seeing this map, therefore, is not isolated—it is part of a larger pattern that has persisted throughout history. Across different cultures and modern UFO research, there have been persistent claims of extraterrestrial activity occurring beneath the Earth's surface. Whether they are called gods, hidden masters, or simply another species that predates our recorded history, the idea of non-human entities residing in underground cities and tunnels is not new.

Take, for example, the Hopi legends of the Ant People. According to Hopi oral tradition, during two great cataclysms, the Ant People sheltered the Hopi underground, saving them from destruction on the surface. These beings were described as having thin limbs, large heads, and telepathic abilities—a description eerily reminiscent of the Greys. The Hopi were led through tunnel systems deep beneath the Earth, where the Ant People cared for them and provided food. Could this story be a distorted memory of extraterrestrial intervention? And if so, does this suggest that underground habitats—like the caverns I was shown—have existed on Earth for thousands of years?

Other ancient cultures tell similar stories of subterranean realms. Hindu texts speak of Patala, a vast underground domain inhabited by the Nagas—serpent-like beings with immense knowledge. In some interpretations, the Nagas were extraterrestrial in origin, possessing technology and wisdom beyond human comprehension. The Tibetan and Buddhist traditions describe Shambhala and Agartha, legendary hidden cities beneath the Earth where enlightened beings reside. These realms were said to be inaccessible to ordinary humans, protected by advanced technology or spiritual barriers—concepts that sound eerily similar to accounts of secret underground alien bases.

The Mayan and Aztec civilizations also spoke of Xibalba, the "Place of Fear"—an underground kingdom inhabited by powerful, god-like beings. This underworld was said to be connected to the surface through hidden tunnels and deep caves. Some researchers have speculated that ancient civilizations had direct contact with beings who lived underground, and that these stories are remnants of real encounters with extraterrestrials.

Even in Western mythology, we find echoes of this theme. The Greek underworld, Hades, was not simply a land of the dead—it was a vast, structured realm beneath the Earth, governed by powerful entities. Many ancient Greeks believed that certain caves and tunnels were gateways to this hidden world, much like how modern UFO researchers describe hidden access points to underground alien bases.

Modern UFOlogy & Underground Alien Bases

In modern UFO research, subterranean bases are a common theme. The most infamous of these is Dulce Base in New Mexico, where whistleblowers claim that hybrid experimentation is occurring beneath the surface. Phil Schneider, a former military engineer, alleged that he witnessed deep underground military bases (DUMBs) where extraterrestrials and human scientists worked together.

Another notable case is Mount Shasta in California, which has long been associated with UFO activity, mystical beings, and stories of an underground civilization. Many locals and visitors have reported strange lights, missing time, and encounters with non-human entities—experiences that parallel abduction accounts.

Bob Lazar, one of the most well-known figures in UFO disclosure, described being briefed on underground installations where extraterrestrials worked with humans on genetic research. He also spoke of massive underground transport systems, suggesting a vast network of hidden tunnels running beneath the United States.

Then there's the "Hollow Earth theory," which—while controversial —suggests that vast subterranean spaces may house ancient extraterrestrial outposts or breakaway civilizations. Some researchers believe that certain deep cave systems remain unexplored because they may lead to active alien or non-human settlements.

Tying This Back to My Experience

If the caverns beneath Illinois are part of this larger phenomenon, then I have to wonder: How many of these installations exist worldwide? Could the Greys be selectively placing these hybrid centers near population hubs, ensuring that they remain close to the genetic material they need? And if these underground chambers aren't just for breeding, but for eventual habitation, what does that say about their long-term plan for the hybrids?

The answers aren't clear, but what is clear is that the map I was shown fits within a much larger historical and modern context. Whether in ancient legends, UFO testimony, or direct encounters like mine, the story is the same: they are here, and many of them are below us.

10

THE DOCTOR WILL TOUCH YOU NOW

By late August 2023, I had been feeling off for months. What started as simple GERD during my courtship with Samantha became something worse. Sharp pains in my stomach had become a near-daily occurrence, flaring up unexpectedly and leaving me in discomfort for hours. Acid reflux had also been plaguing me, not just in my esophagus but throughout my digestive tract, like something was fundamentally wrong inside me. I chalked it up to stress, diet, or maybe just bad luck, but a nagging feeling in the back of my mind told me it was something more.

Despite the discomfort, I had resigned myself to just dealing with it. After all, life doesn't stop for stomach pain. I had other things on my mind—work, responsibilities, and the lingering emotions from my last remembered encounter. The revelation of my hybrid son had stayed with me in ways I hadn't expected. I had spent weeks replaying the moment in my mind, wondering what they weren't telling me. Had they shown him to me as a test? A warning? A taunt?

Whatever the answer, the knowledge that my child was out there, somewhere, had left a mark on me. It wasn't something I could discuss with anyone—not even Samantha, who may have been the boy's mother. And yet, for all the questions I still had about that experience, I wasn't expecting to be taken again so soon.

When the abduction came, I didn't wake in my bed or lying on a strange metal table. Instead, I became aware that I was already standing, my body stiff and disoriented. My first sensation was an uncomfortable one—pressure against my lower abdomen, a warm sensation radiating through my gut. And then, as I blinked into awareness, I realized someone was touching me.

Seated before me was who I believed to be a human doctor and whose hand was cupping my genitals. Just as I began to become aware of my situation and surroundings, my mental fog lifted somewhat as I felt a surge of sensation from the doctor's hand that traveled from my genitals up into my abdomen and kidneys. This sensation aroused my level of consciousness even further where my awareness had peaked as had a sense of annoyance.

"Hey, what are you doing to me?" I protested. "Who are you?" I didn't offer any physical resistance to the uncomfortable sensation of being touched down there, but I had no compulsion against complaining. The 'doctor' said nothing in response to my question, so in the ensuing moments as I awaited some kind of reply, I began to take in my surroundings.

This 'doctor' and I were in a very large room, which I would compare in size to a small warehouse with high ceilings. Perhaps 18 to 20 feet high. The walls and floor, as in previous encounters, were pewter grey and only the immediate area surrounding us was moderately illuminated. As before, no visible source could be discerned for the lighting. Just beyond the perimeter of our area, in the shadows, I could see a dozen or more very tall grays facing our position as though to observe my interactions with the doctor.

"So why did you touch me down there? Where are we? What do you want?" I continued. The doctor stood up from his bench seat and walked past me, toward the center of the room. Turning to follow, I noticed I had been standing in front of a bench seat of my own, which I had nearly stumbled over in my effort to pursue. The doctor walked toward a tall, cylindrical closet at the center of the room. The opening to the closet had to be eight or nine feet tall and a bright light emanated from it in stark contrast to the darkened room. The closet itself seemed to extend in height all the way to the ceiling. While walking toward the closet, I began to act belligerently toward the doctor, as I felt disrespected for his lack of response to my queries. While I have difficulty remembering my exact comments directed at the doctor, my behavior was increasingly rude. After reaching the brightly lit 'closet,' the doctor entered which I presume was to retrieve something he needed. Once he reemerged, something in my awareness changed where I suddenly believed that the doctor who emerged was a different doctor. My visual memory, of course, recalls that it appeared to be the same individual. Perhaps he didn't care for my behavior and used a post hypnotic veil to "reset" my attitude? Proceeding under the assumption that I was speaking to a new doctor, I accompanied him back to the set of benches we had previously occupied. During our walk to the benches, I remember complaining to this new doctor that the 'other doctor' was very rude to me and was touching my "balls" and that I didn't like it. The doctor sat down and invited me to do the same by motioning with his hand.

Upon sitting, the doctor leaned forward toward me and placed both his hands on my abdomen, moving them around in semicircular motions. It was during these moments that I got a better look at this individual. He wasn't like the taller greys or the smaller ones. This individual had a somewhat protruding belly. He didn't wear any clothes, which I had previously not noticed, and his face was chubby. He had large cheeks to go with his very large eyes. If I were to compare his features to something familiar, I'd say he reminded me of a frog. In my entranced state, I was supposed to think he was human, but knew he wasn't. My mind wanted to see this frog-like person in a human way, so he appeared, strangely enough to look like a famous character actor named Wallace Shawn. But that would be inconceivable.

While the doctor had his hands on my abdomen, and as I was attempting to converse with him, I was distracted by the conversations occurring in the back of the room between the dozen or more tall greys observing us. They weren't speaking audibly, mind you, but telepathically amongst themselves. I couldn't understand a thing they were saying, but I could hear every single one of them simultaneously, which filled my mind with chatter that I couldn't filter out in my efforts to speak with the doctor. Increasingly annoyed, I became angry and looked away from the doctor toward our observers standing in the shadows. I didn't know how to tell them to be quiet, as I didn't understand what they were saying to one another, so I used my open, left hand in a downward sweeping motion so as to suggest they be quiet and go away.

Just as I had made this hand gesture, I heard all the chatter between them fall instantly silent. And like some choreographed ensemble, they all turned their backs to us and walked further back into the shadows closer to the wall. I then noticed them turn back to face us and continued their observations. But I couldn't see them clearly any longer.

Moments after this, the doctor removed his hands from my abdomen and raised his head to meet my gaze. "You have an enemy inside you." He said to me, telepathically. In my entranced confusion, I tried to make sense of his words. "An anemone?" I thought to myself, thinking he was speaking the word for "sea urchin." I replayed his words in my mind and realized my mistake.

The doctor continued "but you're going to feel better in a few days." Just as he communicated those last few words, I saw the doctor collapse into a slumped posture with an exhausted, sad look on his face. I don't know if he was sad because I was being rude to him or if he used his own energy to treat some disease that I had and it exhausted him. Part of me suspects both possibilities may be true.

Shortly after witnessing my doctor slump on his bench before me, I lost consciousness. While I don't know what time I was taken, I awoke to see the clock in my bedroom indicated 4:45 a.m.

After opening my eyes, I sat up and grabbed the remote to activate the lights in my room. I turned the red lights on so as not to shock my brain with bright light. As I sat pondering what had occurred, I placed my hands on my belly and realized that my gut felt better than it had in years. The GERD that had plagued me for at least two years was gone, as were the sharp pains in my stomach that I had felt the last fifteen months or so.

"You have an enemy inside you," I recalled the doctor telling me. What could that have meant? Was my GERD something more serious? Eight months prior, shortly after my breakup with my girlfriend Samantha, I learned that she had been diagnosed with stage 2 stomach cancer. And she had developed discomfort in her stomach around the same time that I did the previous year. Could the two be related? Her doctors had biopsied some red, irritated spots in her stomach during an endoscopy and they proved to be cancerous. Her treatment involved cutting out a small portion of her stomach. I am happy to report that this surgery proved to be successful. But could I have had the same thing?

The symptoms I was experiencing for so long were relieved for six or seven months. However, likely due to my lackluster diet, my symptoms of GERD and sharp stomach pains did return by May of 2024. As a result, I chose to consult a GI doctor and he performed a colonoscopy and upper endoscopy. What they found was a nasty H Pylori infection in my stomach. So bad, in fact, he chose to biopsy some red, irritated spots he found. The spots he photographed and biopsied looked nearly identical to the ones Samantha had that proved to be cancerous for her. So this begs my question; was the 'enemy inside' me cancer? Did I acquire the H Pylori infection from Samantha? Or did she acquire that from me? Some cursory research showed me that H Pylori can be transmissible via kissing, so our cases could be related.

If I did briefly have stomach cancer, why did they treat me? Are they ensuring my survival so that I may continue to be a tissue donor for breeding? Did they take Samantha's pregnancy because they detected her cancer and didn't want it to harm the fetus? If that were the case, why wouldn't they treat Samantha? Since they didn't, it seems likely they would have stolen our child either way.

Perhaps there was nothing altruistic about their healing. Maybe I wasn't saved—I was simply maintained. If I am an investment, then my well-being only matters insofar as it serves their goals. This leaves me feeling like a hostage who was given necessary medical care, not out of kindness, but out of utility.

I find myself caught between resentment and reluctant gratitude. Am I truly being watched over, or merely kept in working order? In the end, I may never know.

A Pattern of Healing: Historical Cases of Extraterrestrial Medical Intervention

In the nearly two years since my encounter with the chubby doctor, I wanted to investigate whether my healing was a unique experience among abductees, or if it were relatively common. My reading indicated that the notion of extraterrestrials healing abductees has been documented for decades, with some of the most well-known abduction cases involving reports of sudden physical recoveries, often following medical procedures performed by non-human entities.

One of the most famous accounts of extraterrestrial healing comes from Whitley Strieber, who described an incident in his book *Transformation* (1988) where a mysterious blue beam was directed at his temple by a Grey-like being. He later discovered that a painful lesion he had been dealing with had disappeared. Strieber was left wondering if the procedure was meant to heal him or if something else had been done—just as I found myself questioning whether the Greys healed my stomach out of necessity or self-interest.

Another case that comes to mind is Calvin Parker, one of the two men involved in the 1973 Pascagoula Abduction. During his experience, Parker recalled being subjected to an invasive medical examination aboard the craft. In the weeks following his encounter, Parker's chronic illness mysteriously disappeared. He later speculated that whatever the beings had done to him may have rid his body of an undiagnosed condition. Much like my own experience, he was left with more questions than answers.

One of the most chilling cases comes from Jesse Long, an abductee who claimed that the Greys took him multiple times throughout his life, beginning in childhood. In one of his later experiences, he recalled being subjected to a surgical procedure where a sharp instrument was inserted into his leg. When he awoke the next morning, the wound was completely healed, with only a small scar left behind. However, years later, he underwent surgery on his leg due to unexplained pain, and to his shock, the doctors removed a small, metallic object embedded deep in his tissue—one that was never naturally introduced. Could this be an example of extraterrestrial nanotechnology, used not only for tracking but for monitoring or regulating his body?

Another compelling case is that of Alec Newald, a New Zealander who vanished for ten days in 1989 and later claimed he had been taken to an extraterrestrial civilization where he lived among advanced beings. During his time with them, the entities explained that Earth's atmosphere and diet were highly toxic to human biology, and that they had corrected some of the cellular damage in his body before returning him home. After his experience, Alec reported feeling physically rejuvenated—as if his body had been somehow restored at a molecular level. His story bears striking similarities to cases where abductees return feeling energetically renewed, as if something within them had been adjusted or optimized beyond human medical capability.

And then there's the account of Dr. Roger Leir, a podiatric surgeon who documented the removal of alleged alien implants from abductees. In his book *The Aliens and the Scalpel*, he described cases where abductees had their injuries healed instantly following encounters, leading to speculation that the implants themselves may have been used to monitor, regulate, or even repair their biological functions. If the Greys see us as genetic resources, could they also be maintaining their investments to ensure abductees remain viable for breeding?

Whether their intentions are benevolent or purely pragmatic, the result remains the same—some abductees are healed. But at what cost? And for what purpose? I am left to wonder: was my healing a gift... or simply a means to ensure my continued use?

11

THE ROOM I COULDN'T ENTER

After my August 2023 encounter, I cannot recall any new visits that year. It's possible, if they were still coming for me, that I was kept asleep and not permitted to be conscious. Or perhaps they finally found a method whereby I couldn't remember our encounters. Either way, the question persisted in my mind whether I have more experiences buried somewhere within my subconscious. By December, I had resolved to investigate that possibility - with hypnosis.

In January of 2024, I decided to escalate my investigation into these experiences, which by that point had become less frequent—or perhaps had shifted into unconscious encounters that I could no longer recall. For the previous year, I had been delving deeper into the abduction phenomenon, determined to understand more about what had been happening to me. I started watching various documentaries on streaming services and came across discussions on regressive hypnosis therapy as a tool for abductees like myself.

It made me wonder: Could I recover more memories that I had suppressed? Were there additional details from the 1970s that remained locked away? Could there be encounters from the mid-90s that I had never consciously recalled? Or even within the experiences

I did remember, were there gaps in my awareness—moments that had been obscured? The possibility intrigued me.

Through my research, I became familiar with a number of individuals who specialize in helping people like me. One of them was Barbara Lamb, whom I had seen featured on Ancient Aliens and in the series ETs Among Us. Barbara is a licensed psychotherapist (now retired) who has spent decades working as a hypnotherapist and regression therapist, guiding individuals through past-life regressions and abduction memory retrieval.

With a little sleuthing, I managed to find Barbara's business number and sent her a text message. Within a few hours, she responded warmly, and we began discussing my case. I explained what I hoped to achieve through hypnosis—specifically, whether I could unlock additional memories beyond what I consciously recalled. After a thoughtful conversation, Barbara agreed to see me as a client, and we scheduled my session for January 20th, 2024.

The day before my session, I flew to San Diego from Chicago O'Hare, where I was met by my brother Norman, who drove down from Los Angeles to visit. We checked into a hotel for my one-night stay, and that evening, I spent four hours recounting my encounters to him in detail. I was grateful for his patience and open-mindedness—receptive ears can be hard to find when discussing something so far outside the average person's frame of reference. But Norman had always had an interest in UFOs and the space program, and perhaps that was part of why he had pursued a career in aerospace as an airframe and powerplant mechanic for United Airlines.

The following morning, after breakfast, we made our way to Barbara Lamb's home office, where she conducts her sessions. My appointment was scheduled for 11:00 a.m., and we arrived fifteen minutes early. After a warm greeting and some brief conversation, my brother excused himself so Barbara and I could begin.

I laid down on a comfortable couch in a softly lit room, the air faintly scented with sage or lavender—something calming. Barbara sat nearby, her voice gentle and precise, guiding me through a progressive relaxation sequence. She spoke slowly, carefully, helping me release the tension in my legs, then my arms, and finally my chest and jaw. With each passing minute, I felt more physically still, as though I were sinking into the fabric of the couch itself.

But inside my mind, a kind of quiet vigilance remained.

Her voice invited me to move backward in time—to recall specific encounters, to gently notice if any details surfaced that I hadn't remembered before. I tried to surrender to the flow of memory, to let impressions rise. I followed her lead with trust, willing to go wherever the session might take me. But even as I drifted into a calm, suggestible state, I became aware of something I hadn't anticipated: a kind of mental stubbornness, as if a gatekeeper had stepped forward within me. I wasn't fighting Barbara. I wasn't resisting her voice. But something inside me wasn't budging.

There were moments when I felt the edge of something—a flicker of color, a whisper of motion, like a half-formed dream—but each time I reached for it, it dissolved. The deeper I tried to go, the more elusive the impressions became. My breathing was slow, my muscles still, but my inner world felt... insulated. Like a room with no windows.

I remember saying aloud, "I feel like I'm standing in front of a door, but I can't open it." She asked me what the door looked like, but I couldn't see one. I just sensed it. Not visually, not even emotionally—just architecturally, as if the architecture of my mind had designed this feature: a sealed room with no handle.

Barbara reassured me that this was okay. That I was doing just fine. And I believed her. Still, I couldn't help but feel a quiet wave of disappointment forming beneath the surface. I had come all this way—physically, emotionally, even financially—to try and unlock something I had suspected for decades was just out of reach. And now, here I was, lying in a peaceful room with a trusted guide, and I couldn't find the way through.

That disappointment softened into reflection as I sat quietly after the session, processing what had just occurred. I hadn't uncovered new memories, but I had discovered something important: that my subconscious might not be unwilling—it might simply be unready. And if so, the question then became: Why?

Was this resistance something I had built myself? Or was it put there by design—either by the greys, or by some deeper mechanism of psychological protection?

It wouldn't be until much later—over a year afterward—that I began to understand the shape of that question more clearly. In April of 2025, during a second hypnosis session with a different practitioner, I discovered that I carried something I hadn't expected: fear. A sharp, instinctive fear tied to the possibility of recovering memories from the period in my childhood when the orbs first began to appear. The realization surprised me. I hadn't felt afraid of those early experiences in a long time—at least not consciously. But there it was, lurking beneath the surface: not just silence, but avoidance. My own subconscious didn't want to look.

And that, perhaps, is why the room wouldn't open. Not because it was empty, but because something in me still feared what might be inside. The memories may exist. The impressions may still be there. But memory is a two-way street. If the mind resists access—even subtly—then recovery becomes an act of courage, not just procedure.

I had hoped that hypnosis would grant me access to something hidden—a room in my mind that I've never been able to enter. But it remained locked. Whether by my own design or by someone else's, I don't yet know. All I know is that I knocked, and the door didn't open.

But that doesn't mean it never will.

I left the session feeling disappointed but not discouraged. Hypnosis does not work the same way for everyone, and I had no reason to doubt Barbara's skill or experience. If anything, my difficulty in accessing deeper memories said more about me than about the process itself. Some people are simply less hypnotizable than others, and I've often found that my mind resists outside influence. Perhaps I'm too analytical—or perhaps I've simply trained myself, consciously or not, to maintain control. But after what I discovered later, I began to wonder if it wasn't logic or willpower standing in the way, but fear. Fear of what might surface if I let go completely.

Whatever the reason, I would not give up. If I couldn't recover these memories through one method of hypnosis, then I would have to find another way.

I've since come to realize that my experience isn't unusual. Others who've walked this path before me—people with their own histories of contact—have described similar challenges when attempting to recover buried memories through hypnosis. Whitley Strieber, in *Communion*, wrote candidly about the uncertainty hypnosis brought into his life. While it helped him recall more than he consciously knew, it also left him unsettled. He often questioned whether the images he retrieved were authentic memories or a hypnotically induced narrative—and admitted that even after the sessions, he still couldn't be sure what was real. The process didn't give him clarity—it deepened the mystery.

Budd Hopkins, whose groundbreaking work *Missing Time* helped shape public understanding of abduction phenomena, also recognized the limits of hypnosis. While he believed strongly in its value, he documented many cases where subjects encountered emotional resistance—what he sometimes referred to as "hitting a wall." Some people simply couldn't go deeper. Others would begin to recover memories, only to be overwhelmed by anxiety or confusion before anything concrete could surface. In his view, it wasn't always about willingness. Sometimes, the mind shut the door all on its own.

David Jacobs, in *The Threat*, took it further. He believed the greys themselves had a hand in preventing full recall. According to Jacobs, abductees often carry "screen memories"—false overlays designed to mask the true nature of what happened. And even under hypnosis, these screen memories can persist. He argued that the visitors were capable of such advanced mental manipulation that traditional methods like regression might only skim the surface. For some experiencers, hypnosis didn't uncover the truth. It merely revealed the layers of interference keeping the truth out of reach.

Hearing this from people who've studied or endured similar phenomena brings a strange kind of relief. I'm not alone in my resistance. My subconscious barrier isn't necessarily a failure of the method—or of my willingness. It might simply be evidence of how deep the conditioning goes. Whether installed by the greys, or developed through years of internal shielding, the result is the same: a mind that won't surrender easily, even when asked to.

And so I remind myself, again, that the room may still be there. The memories may still be waiting. But it might take something more than hypnosis to find the key.

Sometimes I think that room in my mind—the one I couldn't enter—was never meant to be forced open. That it isn't a vault with a key, but more like a seed beneath soil, waiting for the right conditions to stir. Maybe memory isn't something to be pried loose, but something that chooses to bloom when it's ready.

And maybe that's what the greys understand about us. Maybe that's why their influence feels so surgical. Not because they're cruel —but because they know how tightly we cling to pain. How much we hide even from ourselves. If they've built walls inside us, they've done so with precise knowledge of where our minds fracture. But if I built that wall myself—if the fear I carry was self-imposed—then the only way through is by walking gently toward it.

For now, I accept that I don't have access to everything. And that's okay. Healing doesn't come all at once, and truth rarely arrives on command. But I've begun the journey. I've knocked on the door. I've sat with the silence. And maybe, in time, I'll hear something stir behind it.

If that moment comes, I'll be ready. Or perhaps, more truthfully, I'll be as ready as I'm allowed to be. Because readiness may not be mine to define. Not entirely. I can knock. I can ask. I can prepare my body, calm my mind, open my heart. But if the greys still hold the lock... if part of my memory belongs to them... then all I can do is wait for the next time they leave something behind. A taste. A sound. A thread. Something to follow. Until then, I'll keep the door in view —and the light on.

12

A TASTE LEFT BEHIND

After meeting with Barbara Lamb, I returned to every day life and routine concerns. Going to work during the week, or visiting my daughter or my parents on weekends. By the month of March, I was preparing to do some home renovations, including painting my living room, dining room, hallway and my daughter's vacant room. I was eager to make the house look nicer, and hoped that my daughter would notice how I fixed up her bedroom and gave her a new queen bed with a padded leather headboard. Before she had moved into her group home, I would often find her hanging out in my bedroom, sitting up in my bed and leaning against its padded headboard as she listened to music on her iPad - her favorite activity. Now, when she would visit home for the occasional weekend sleep-over, she could enjoy her own bed - just as nice as daddy's. The thought of seeing the excitement in her mannerisms motivated me to accomplish this project in a timely fashion.

On a Friday night in mid-March, 2024 the evening before I was to begin my painting project, I decided to watch a movie to relax and fixed myself an Old Fashioned cocktail, with bourbon - my new favorite drink. Over the previous 18 months, I had enjoyed an Old Fashioned on the occasional weekend, sometimes two or three times in a month. On this particular evening, it had been two weeks since I had my previous nightcap. But tonight, I was treating myself. So I made a smoked old fashioned, using oak wood chips... and garnished my elixir with a thin slice of orange rind and some brandied cherries, spiced with cinnamon and anise. As I watched a rented movie in my living room, I felt mellowed and content. And after finishing my drink, fixed a second one. By the time I had finished the movie, my second Old Fashioned had been thoroughly dispatched and I was ready for bed, feeling drowsy and slightly inebriated. I didn't have a care in the world, except for the anticipation of painting the next day.

I fell fast asleep around 11:00 pm. I don't remember having any dreams during the period I was asleep, but I do remember waking up. In a strange room.

I don't know what time it was, but I awoke in a reclined, sitting position. As though I had been placed in a chair with a seat back that tilted backwards by 25 or 30 degrees. This time, the room I was in wasn't pewter grey as in previous encounters... the walls were white. And the room was brightly lit, uncharacteristic of so many dimly-lit rooms in which I had awakened, previously.

Surrounding me were three tall greys. I couldn't see their feet, as I perceived my seat was raised a few feet on a platform of some kind. I could see them from the waist, up. I had considerable difficulty making sense of my surroundings and the situation, as I was still somewhat inebriated. So while I was fighting their usual entrancement, I was also feeling the effects of the bourbon.

They were upset with me. I could feel that. Most of their words scrambled in my mind. I couldn't understand their communication this time around. Was it the alcohol? Was it affecting the telepathy? Just as I had the thought that I wasn't in the best condition to interact with them, I finally perceived some intelligible English. "You shouldn't drink alcohol."

As I had been rude and annoyed with them in previous encounters, their suggestion and visible disappointment with me triggered my irritation. I genuinely disliked being taken from my home, controlled and being unable to resist or even communicate on my own terms. These people! They never respected me. While I didn't have these specific thoughts at that exact moment, that was the motivation behind my disdain. That was my mindset.

"Hey, fuck you!" I said, verbally. "I haven't had a drink since two weeks ago Thursday!" At that moment, the two greys directly facing me turned their heads to exchange knowing, displeased glances. And the one to the right gave a nod to the other. What was that about?

I lost consciousness after my terse retort, as I'm certain they didn't want to engage in further discourse. I awoke later that morning, a little after 5:00 am. Sitting up in bed, I searched my memory - desperately, trying to make sense of what just occurred. Why did they take me this time? Harvesting semen? Bone marrow? A health checkup? I had no clue. All I could remember is that they were upset that I had consumed alcohol. "Who cares?" I thought. I don't drink enough to be considered an addict. I don't hang out at pubs. And the occasional bourbon isn't going to hurt my health, is it?

I decided to let it go and not bother me. It was Saturday and I had to get to Home Depot as early as possible to retrieve some additional supplies needed for the day's painting. I wanted to purchase additional canvas drop cloths and some extra paint roller refills and a roll of three-inch, blue masking tape.

Over the next two weekends, I managed to complete all the rooms I intended to paint. I had blocked off my AirBnB schedule for two weeks, so I could work without inconveniencing my guests, or myself. I even did some painting after work on a few week days. On the day I had finished, it occurred to me I should reward myself with another old fashioned. I hadn't had one since a few Fridays prior, and it would be a welcome respite to my final day's toils. After cleaning up and tidying all the work areas in the house, I had put away the equipment and the leftover paint - stowing them on shelves in the garage. I was ready to relax.

Setting up my cocktail supplies on the island counter in the kitchen, I poured two and a half shots of bourbon, two shakes of bitters, added simple syrup and sliced my orange rind - which I speared along with a few brandied cherries. I covered the bourbon with my smoking kit, fired the oak chips with my butane torch and watched with anticipation as the wood smoke lowered into the glass, infusing its wonderful aroma into the bourbon. I topped this divine ambrosia off with ice. I was going to enjoy this!

Or so I thought.

Retreating to the living room, I reclined in my easy chair, Old Fashioned in hand and settled into another rented movie. This time, however, something was "off." The Old Fashioned tasted normally. It was consistent with any other I had made, or enjoyed at my favorite restaurants. But this time, it tasted weird to me. I just didn't like it. After several sips, there was something vile about it. For reasons I couldn't explain, I hated it.

I set my glass down, staring at the liquid as if it had betrayed me. It wasn't the bourbon itself—it was me. The taste hadn't changed, yet something inside me had. Had they done something to me? I ran through the possibilities in my mind. I knew my body, and I knew my habits. I wasn't a heavy drinker. I had never struggled with alcohol, nor had I ever had any reason to give it up. And yet, here I was, recoiling from a drink I had once savored. It wasn't a matter of preference—it was a visceral rejection.

I couldn't shake the thought: Had the Greys altered something in me? Maybe it wasn't just their disapproval—maybe they had acted on it. Had they implanted a suggestion, a post-hypnotic aversion to alcohol? Or had they somehow changed my physiology, tweaking some neurological switch so that the very act of drinking now repelled me?

Or was it simpler than that?

Was I just remembering what it felt like to be under their scrutiny? To feel their disappointment radiate through me, their silent command sinking into my subconscious? Maybe the thought of drinking had become tangled up in my resentment toward them. A violation of my autonomy, one more thing they had taken from me without my consent. And yet, the strangest thing was, I didn't mind.

Whatever the cause—whether psychological conditioning, a biological alteration, or something even stranger—I had no desire to fight it. It didn't feel like a loss. I simply... no longer cared for drinking. The appeal was gone, as if it had never belonged to me in the first place.

The Old Fashioned sat untouched for the rest of the night, and the next day, I poured it down the drain. That was the last time I ever made one.

Whatever happened in that bright, sterile room... it stayed with me.

The Programming That Sticks

In the days that followed my last remembered encounter, I couldn't stop thinking about what had changed. Not just that I didn't want an Old Fashioned anymore—but that something in me didn't want it. It wasn't willpower. It wasn't a decision. It was reflexive, like a switch had been thrown.

I had heard about screen memories and blocked recollections before. But this felt different. This wasn't about forgetting. This was about modifying behavior—like some kind of post-hypnotic suggestion that had been embedded in my mind during the encounter, only now revealing itself in my daily life.

I began digging deeper into the work of others who had studied the phenomenon—researchers like Derrel Sims and Barbara Lamb —people who had worked directly with abductees over many years. What I found startled me.

Derrel Sims, known for his focus on physical evidence and implants, also documented behavioral shifts in his cases—sudden changes in preference, unexplained phobias, and abrupt lifestyle corrections that mirrored my own. One of his clients, he wrote, abruptly stopped drinking alcohol—just stopped, overnight—with no prior struggle or intent to quit. The man had simply lost all interest. In other cases, Sims described people who developed aversions to specific sounds, foods, or even colors after encounters—none of which they could explain. Sims speculated that some of these responses might be induced neurologically, others psychologically— but all of them had the flavor of deep behavioral programming.

Barbara Lamb, in her extensive regression work with abductees, echoed similar patterns. She reported multiple clients who experienced sudden, drastic shifts in diet, lifestyle, or emotional habits after encounters. Some became more spiritual. Others found themselves inexplicably drawn to certain locations or activities. A few even lost interest in longtime hobbies or habits, without ever connecting it to the encounter—until regression brought the link to light. Lamb believed that in some cases, the visitors had installed post-hypnotic suggestions—commands or conditions that would activate later, silently guiding the abductee's choices without conscious awareness.

And then there are the many unnamed cases—those catalogued by Budd Hopkins, David Jacobs, and Whitley Strieber—where abductees not only lost memories of the events but also found themselves behaving differently in their aftermath. Quiet, almost imperceptible changes that often didn't register as significant until much later.

Looking at all this, I can't help but wonder: was my revulsion toward alcohol truly my own? Or was it gifted—or rather, installed—by them?

If the Greys can erase memories, induce paralysis, and communicate telepathically, is it really so far-fetched to think they can rewire preferences, eliminate cravings, or plant aversions?

And more importantly—what else have they changed in me that I haven't noticed yet?

These patterns weren't isolated. Across the broader abduction literature, other researchers have touched on the possibility of post-hypnotic influence—not just in how we remember, but in how we behave.

Budd Hopkins, in *Missing Time* and *Witnessed*, noted subtle psychological shifts in his subjects—unexplained changes in their emotional demeanor, daily habits, and sometimes their social relationships. Several abductees found themselves withdrawing from friendships or changing career paths shortly after major encounters. Others developed sudden compulsions to alter their diets or remove certain environmental triggers from their homes. While Hopkins focused primarily on memory retrieval and physical evidence, he acknowledged the unconscious behavioral drift that often followed close contact.

David Jacobs, who spent decades conducting hypnotic regressions, went further. He suggested that abductees were often conditioned—not only to forget, but to comply. In *The Threat* and *Walking Among Us*, Jacobs described a growing trend among abductees to feel resigned, as though some part of them had been subdued. His work with so-called "hubrids"—hybrid beings placed in human society—raised another disturbing possibility: that abductees might be programmed to assist or remain passive in the face of an unfolding integration agenda. If true, then sudden behavioral shifts—such as changes in intimacy, parenting, or lifestyle—may not just be side effects. They could be the goal.

And then there's Whitley Strieber, who never shied away from the emotional and existential complexity of his own encounters. In *Transformation*, he detailed a period where he found himself consumed by guilt, emotional withdrawal, and spiritual longing—none of which aligned with his normal self. He wondered if his visitors had reconfigured his inner world, not just his memories. In later interviews and writings, he speculated that certain abductees were being altered from within, their minds quietly tuned to new frequencies of behavior or perception, often without their knowledge.

These aren't tidy, cinematic revelations. They're slow leaks—shifts in thought and instinct that don't announce themselves with flashing lights or eerie music. They slip beneath the surface, unnoticed until one day, something simple—a drink you used to enjoy, a desire you no longer feel, a reflex you no longer question—falls away. And when you look for the reason, you realize... you didn't make that choice. It was made for you.

That's the flavor of control. And it lingers.

13

THE TRANSPARENT MIND

In chapter 12, "A Taste Left Behind," I discussed how encounters with the greys can leave lasting impressions upon one's psyche, not the least of which is behavioral modification imposed via post hypnotic suggestion or similar mechanism. As I looked back upon my life and examine who I have been and became, I started to reflect on how much of my persona may have been influenced by my interactions with them.

While I can only confidently point to three major periods of my life where I suspect prolonged contact - The early 1970's, the early to mid 1990's and the early to mid 2020's - it nonetheless seems apparent that these intervals were more than adequate to effect genuine changes. Particularly, I suspect, in my youth - where deep impressions can shape a person during their most formative years of development.

During my most recent flap of encounters, it became painfully obvious to me that the greys can seize control not only over one's body - which was a powerful and articulated type of control - but also over one's mind. When I communicated with the greys via the sign over my bed, alerting them to my awareness of their presence, they immediately investigated how I knew. When I awoke to find Syczylick hovering on top of me, and we touched foreheads, my mind became an open book for his perusal. When I awoke during subsequent encounters, my mind was prone to suggestion regarding what I saw, where screen memories would imprint upon the experience, with the intention that I would misremember the encounters and dismiss them - confusing them with dreams.

These experiences impress me, in as much that I realize that no shadowed corner of my mind appears to be hidden from them - if they need to know anything about me that suits their agenda. In short, there's never been an incentive or opportunity to conceal anything when I was in their presence. While I do not remember seeing greys as a toddler, that does not mean I don't possess some repressed memories of them. And during this four-year period from 1970-1974, could their forays into my mind - as a means to lessen my trauma - have affected my personality, even in subtle ways?

Throughout my childhood, I had a reputation of openness among my family and peers. I shared everything. Sometimes to the point of oversharing - when it was usually and completely unnecessary. This created a social dynamic, however, where my lack of mystery among my peers became a reason for disinterest. That became a constant source of isolation for me. While I had plenty of friends, those who were closest to me had to exercise a level of patience, knowing that this trait of mine was something I could not help. And in my mind, when I would connect with a person, I had this kind of need for efficiency - a tendency to offer large information-dumps, as though I were catching the person up to speed on a topic or project. And this was something I commonly did in my youth. While I have largely outgrown this tendency, and exercise more patience while socializing, I would call my evolution more of a learned behavior. My brain would prefer information-dumps when communicating what it knows. Why is that?

In my life as an autism parent, I have learned that many parents of autistic children can be considered slightly within the spectrum themselves - some earning a diagnosis of "Asperger's syndrome," - which usually follows an evaluation that was performed because of a need for a subsequent treatment - usually some pharmaceutical intervention. However in my life, no such evaluation, diagnosis or treatment was ever necessary. I have lived a perfectly functional, if not entirely normal, life. Despite that, I understand that the traits I outlined from my youth could fit within the category of Asperger's. So why bring it up? Why make this a topic in the memoir? Aren't these traits satisfied entirely by this syndrome?

In the absence of any other context, I'd be inclined to agree. But in my life, there is another context. A presence and an influence that has a profound ability to manipulate memory and behaviors. A force that related and communicated to me in similar fashion - immediate and impressed information dumps as though one computer were exchanging files with another.

And maybe that's the connection. Maybe, over time, I internalized this model of communication. When I cared about someone, or felt a rapport forming, I wanted to "download" everything relevant at once. I wasn't being performative or seeking validation. It simply felt efficient. Like I needed to orient the other person before we could continue. Like the act of withholding, or spacing things out, was somehow dishonest.

This mirrored how the greys communicated with me: not through speech, not even through images alone, but through total transmission—intention, memory, emotional context, all at once, sometimes without warning. That kind of exposure is difficult to describe. It isn't like having a conversation; it's more like having a part of yourself excavated, inspected, and returned to you in altered form.

So I wonder—if my behavioral openness isn't simply a trait or social quirk, could it be residue? A reflection of how I was interacted with repeatedly throughout my life? Perhaps a psychological adaptation to repeated psychic invasions, where my mind was laid bare over and over again, until the idea of privacy itself began to erode.

It would explain why, for most of my life, I've felt no incentive to hold things back. My brothers could keep secrets; I struggled to. They could compartmentalize; I preferred to spill everything at once.

Maybe I wasn't just being "open." Maybe I was trying to preempt the inevitable. To get ahead of it. To confess before I could be exposed.

I've often thought of Whitley Strieber in this context. In *Communion*, he writes not only about the trauma of his experiences, but the deeply unsettling realization that his inner world was not private. He speaks of being observed—not just physically, but psychically—and of the compulsion to share, to confess, to lay everything bare in the face of a force that already knew everything anyway. In a later work, he asked aloud whether the visitors had "infected" his mind with the need to speak, as if they'd implanted not just memories, but a mandate.

Jim Sparks, too, described something eerily similar in his book *The Keepers: An Alien Message for the Human Race*. After years of intense, conscious interaction with nonhuman beings, Sparks developed a sense of being used—not in the physical sense alone, but as a kind of conduit. He wrote about experiencing direct "downloads" of information and being tasked with relaying messages, often against his will. His emotional transparency became raw, even unfiltered, as though the usual boundaries between inner and outer life had dissolved. It wasn't just that he wanted to speak—it was as if he had to, as though he were broadcasting rather than conversing.

What I share with these men isn't just experience—it's aftermath. The psychic ripple. The behavioral fingerprint left behind by those who never ask, but always take.

I suppose this is why writing a memoir like this feels less like a decision and more like a compulsion. It's as if I'm finishing a conversation that started long ago—one in which my responses were never requested, only extracted. But now, for once, I'm choosing the words. I'm laying the pages open on *my own terms*.

Betty Andreasson, whose deeply spiritual encounters are chronicled in *The Andreasson Affair* by Raymond E. Fowler, also illustrates this phenomenon. Her experiences with the beings—described as both robotic and angelic—often involved direct telepathic communication. But more than that, she seemed to embrace a kind of radical vulnerability after her experiences. In interviews and transcripts,

Andreasson speaks without hesitation or reservation, often sharing personal, symbolic visions and metaphysical insights that most people would guard carefully. There's a purity to her transparency, as though the repeated exposure to these beings had stripped away any instinct to withhold. What stood out was not just her belief in what happened, but her complete willingness to share it—all of it—with strangers, researchers, and the public. She did not seem embarrassed by the spiritual strangeness or the deeply personal nature of her revelations. In fact, she seemed unable—or perhaps unwilling—to separate her inner experience from the outer world anymore.

There's something hauntingly familiar about that.

To live without mental privacy isn't just about what's taken from you—it's about what's reshaped within you. I don't remember ever consciously deciding to be open with people. I just was. As if my inner world, already breached by something I could never quite name, had learned that secrets were an illusion. And once the illusion shattered, it never quite reformed.

It's not that I lacked boundaries, or didn't want them. It's that somewhere along the line, the part of me that might have naturally protected its inner life... gave up. Whether as a defense mechanism, or an unconscious adaptation to the frequent invasions of mind and memory, I found myself becoming someone who preemptively discloses. I offer the contents of my mind to others almost automatically, as if to say, Here, take it before someone else does.

And while I have grown more reserved with age, the reflex remains.

I've often wondered what kind of person I might have become in a life untouched by such forces. Would I have been more guarded? Would I have learned to cultivate mystery, to keep a part of myself protected from others? Or was this transparency always in me—and the encounters merely amplified it, weaponized it, or perhaps even hijacked it?

But now, as I write these pages, something has shifted. For the first time in my life, I'm not just sharing out of reflex—I'm doing so with intention. I am the one laying down the narrative. I am the one choosing which thoughts to show and which ones to shape into sentences. There's a strange empowerment in that. I can feel the old instinct rising—just tell everything, all at once—but now, I get to decide what stays and what gets spoken. Not because I have anything to hide, but because I finally have something to author.

This memoir, then, is not just the act of telling my story. It is an act of reclamation. A quiet rebellion against years of psychological transparency I never consented to. For once, I am speaking on my own terms. And if I choose to open the door fully, it will be because I hold the key.

Of all the areas in my life where this pattern of radical openness has made itself known, none have been more affected than my love life. In friendships, this trait could be softened by time—people got to know me gradually, through shared experience. Over weeks or years, they came to understand that my openness wasn't performative, and certainly not manipulative. It stemmed from a place of warmth, sincerity, and a desire to connect. Those who stuck around saw the reciprocal generosity that came with it—both materially and in spirit.

But dating? That was different.

First impressions carry disproportionate weight in romantic settings, and my habit of oversharing—particularly in my twenties, late thirties, and well into my forties—had a way of setting off alarms. It wasn't just that I talked too much; it was what I talked about. Deep personal experiences, emotional impressions, metaphysical questions, or ideas that belonged to a far more intimate stage of connection—I would lay these things out early, sometimes unconsciously. To me, it felt natural. Honest. Efficient, even. But to someone sitting across the table from me on a first date, it could feel overwhelming. Or worse, strange.

There were times when I could feel the retreat happening in real time. The subtle shift in posture, the careful recalibration of tone, the polite attempt to steer the conversation back to surface-level normalcy. And while I'd occasionally catch myself and try to ease back, the moment had already done its damage. The mystery was gone. And with it, sometimes, the interest.

In hindsight, I can't fault those women. They were responding to a presentation of self that felt… unguarded in a way that most people aren't prepared for. In a world where trust is earned incrementally, I was trying to hand over the whole package in one sitting. Not out of desperation, but because that's how my inner world functioned. That's how I had come to understand connection.

It wasn't until much later in life—well into my mid-40s—that I learned to temper this instinct. To let people arrive at their own pace, rather than rush to meet them at the finish line. That restraint was not instinctual; it was learned. And if I'm being honest, it still feels unnatural at times. Like holding back a wave that wants to crash forward. But I've come to see the value in it. Some connections are stronger when they're allowed to build slowly. When revelation becomes a gift, not a flood.

Still, I wonder how many of those early moments were shaped not just by my personality, but by the imprint of something deeper. If my tendency to "lay it all out" came from the part of me that had long since surrendered to exposure—whose mind had been turned inside-out by something that never asked for permission—then maybe those awkward moments weren't just social missteps. Maybe they were echoes.

There's a strange kind of grief in realizing you've never truly had a private interior life—not because you willingly shared it, but because it was accessed before you had the words to defend it. When I think about the idea of mental privacy, I don't think of secrets. I think of stillness. Of the right to carry a thought, or a question, or a pain, without needing to hand it over. And I think of how rare that has been for me. How easily my inner life seems to have been read, either by the beings I encountered or by the learned reflex that tells me to volunteer it all before someone goes looking.

Even now, as I write this chapter, I feel the familiar pull—not just to be honest, but to be utterly honest. To peel back every layer. It's a kind of compulsion, yes—but also a strange form of penance. If I was invaded, if I was read without consent, then maybe the only way to reclaim agency is to step forward and say: Here. I'll show you. But it will be my choice this time. Maybe that's what this memoir really is. A reclamation of boundaries, even as I seem to erase them. A paradox I've learned to live with.

Because here's the truth: I don't believe I'll ever be the kind of person who holds back completely. The wiring feels too old, too baked in. But I've learned to recognize the difference between being transparent out of habit... and being transparent out of courage. One is conditioned. The other is chosen. And perhaps there's something quietly powerful about owning a mind that's been laid bare—and still insisting on authorship. Still shaping the story.

In a life touched by forces that have never asked permission, I've finally learned to say: This is mine. And if I share it with you, it will be because I have chosen to. Not because I was compelled. That, to me, is the true definition of healing. Not forgetting. Not even protecting. But choosing the shape of your own exposure.

In recent years, I've started telling my story not just in words, but in images. Recreating key moments through 3D illustrations has become another outlet for the same instinct that's shaped so much of my life: the desire to communicate everything all at once. In a way, each illustration functions like an information-dump in visual form—an efficient transfer of feeling, atmosphere, and memory without the delay or limitations of verbal explanation. Where language must unfold line by line, an image lands immediately. This is why I feel such urgency to create them. They are not just expressions—they are transmissions.

And they serve another purpose. In these visual reconstructions, I'm not just recalling the events—I'm shaping them. I choose the lighting, the angles, the expressions. It's an act of authorship, but also of emotional confrontation. Sometimes, I'll feel a rush of anxiety when a scene starts to look too accurate—too familiar. But that anxiety tells me I'm getting close to something true.

I think of these images as part of the same process that brought me to this memoir. They are artifacts of autonomy. They allow me to say: You may have taken something from me, but I am taking it back —frame by frame, word by word. And perhaps most importantly, they remind me that the mind they once walked through uninvited… now has doors. And I am the one who opens them.

This chapter, like so many others in this book, is an artifact of that choice. A glimpse into the transparent mind—but offered now with intention, not surrender.

I sometimes wonder how many others carry this same subtle fracture and never question its origin. How many people feel the impulse to share too much, too soon—believing it's just a quirk, or a flaw, or poor social instinct—when in fact, it might be something deeper. A pattern learned through contact. A survival response masquerading as personality. We tend to think of trauma in terms of what it takes away, but it also leaves behind strange gifts. And in my case, it left me with this: a transparent mind, shaped by forces that never asked for permission—but now choosing, moment by moment, what to reveal and what to protect. Not because I'm broken. But because I remember what it feels like to be laid bare without a voice. And now, the voice is mine.

14

MUFON AND THE MEDIA FLAP

After March of 2024, I don't recall any additional encounters with certainty. There were times, during the rest of the year, when I had occasion to suspect I may have been visited. While I didn't experience any vivid dreams involving the greys or wake up in strange places, I had emotional impressions that made me feel I hadn't slept normally. Just the impression of contact. A mere whisper from my subconscious — like the melody of a song you can't name — but not enough to be certain.

By November of 2024, I decided to reach out to the broader UFO community to see if my case might garner any interest. After some research online, I came across the website of MUFON — the Mutual UFO Network. On their site, they offered a form specifically for reporting an "abduction or non-human contact." I clicked the link and completed the contact and survey forms. Within a few days, I received an email from a field investigator assigned to Illinois, named Timothy Aines. After a brief exchange, we arranged to do a Zoom interview.

On the day of our interview, Timothy and I spoke for several hours. I shared as many details about my experiences as I could — beginning with the most extraordinary encounters and eventually filling in the lesser but still meaningful ones. I also showed him the illustrations I had created using 3D CGI software. These weren't simple sketches; they were immersive recreations of what I saw, built with great care and attention to lighting, composition, and atmosphere. Timothy appreciated the value of those images, not just as visual aids, but as a record of memory — snapshots of a reality few people can imagine.

Creating those images was never just about accuracy. It was about memory. The scenes I chose to reconstruct weren't random—they were the ones that haunted me the most. The ones I kept circling back to at night, trying to understand. I would pose figures in a 3D workspace, adjusting limb angles, eye direction, proximity, lighting, until something inside me said: Yes. That's it. That's what I saw.

And sometimes, in that process, new details would surface. A gesture I hadn't remembered. A color that felt suddenly, inexplicably right. It was as if the act of recreating the scene reopened the memory, not unlike a dream returning in fragments after you wake up. I wasn't just illustrating—I was decoding.

The lighting was always important. Many of these encounters took place in dim or dreamlike environments, and I found that soft edge lighting, low contrast, or even exaggerated ambient glow helped match what I had seen. It wasn't photorealism I was chasing—it was emotional realism. A way to transmit not just the image, but the feeling of the moment.

One of the hardest scenes I ever created was the one we ended up using for the cover—Syczylick on top of me, our foreheads touching, my hand pressed to his shoulder. Recreating that image meant recreating *him*—his size, his posture, the eerie calm of his presence. I stared at that face for hours, refining the subtle tilt of his head, the strange anatomy of his collarbone, the way his eyes watched without blinking. It was as intimate as it was disturbing.

Another scene that left me emotionally shaken was the one with the grey doctor—his hands placed gently but authoritatively on my abdomen. There was something profoundly violating in that moment, not because it was violent, but because it was so clinical.

Like I was no longer a person, just a specimen he was assessing. That encounter left a residue I still can't fully explain.

And yet, despite those moments, it was the garage encounter that hit me the hardest. Not because it was the most complex to render—but because it was burned into me. That scene, more than any other, shattered the wall of doubt I still carried about my 1994 experience. Waking up in that position, paralyzed, under their control—it wasn't just frightening. It was clarifying. It was the moment I knew: this was real. It had always been real. And every pixel of that scene felt like a jolt of that truth.

To see those illustrations appreciated—not just by MUFON investigators, but later - by television producers—felt validating. These weren't just personal artifacts anymore. They were becoming part of the public record. Part of a broader visual language for a phenomenon too often dismissed as fantasy. And for once, I didn't have to explain it all with words. The images spoke for themselves.

After recording my testimony and uploading my illustrations to MUFON's records, Timothy told me that he considered my case among the top five he had encountered. He also noted that MUFON receives approximately 8,000 cases each year — between UFO sightings and abduction reports — a reminder of just how many people come forward, even if few ever make headlines. He informed me that he planned to petition MUFON leadership to allow him to present my case at the 2025 MUFON Symposium. After a committee vote, it was selected as the first of four cases to be featured in a presentation titled "Best of the ERT" — a reference to MUFON's Experiencer Resource Team.

After our initial round of calls and emails, I made the decision in December of 2024 to begin writing this memoir. I started during the second weekend of December and committed myself fully to the task, with the goal of completing the manuscript by June 2025. If the symposium led to any kind of public interest, I wanted the book ready by the month before — hoping it might attract a publisher.

January 2025

The very next month, Timothy contacted me again to let me know that the production team behind Ancient Aliens was seeking new experiencer cases for an upcoming episode in their 21st season. A committee of ten MUFON senior staff members had selected five cases to refer to the show's producers, and mine was one of them. I agreed to participate if chosen and waited while MUFON submitted my case summary to Prometheus Entertainment, the show's production company.

By January 15th, I was contacted by their producers and invited to participate in a recorded Zoom interview as part of their selection process. A young associate producer named Nuria conducted the interview, which lasted about an hour and fifteen minutes. Based on that conversation, I was later sent an official invitation to appear on the show.

The moment I received the email confirming my inclusion on Ancient Aliens, I had to read it twice. It felt surreal. For the past five years, I had watched the show religiously — not just for entertainment, but as a form of education. It had been my self-guided curriculum in all things extraterrestrial: historical visitations, government coverups, hybrid programs, and especially the abduction phenomenon. The people featured on the show were voices I had come to recognize and respect. To go from anonymous viewer to featured subject felt like stepping through the screen.

I sat with that feeling for a while — part disbelief, part validation. For so long, I had kept my experiences to myself, unsure how they would be received, unsure even what to call them. And now, a show I once watched in private was reaching back through the television and saying: You belong here.

On January 26th, 2025, I flew to Los Angeles, spent the night at a hotel, and was taken to the filming set the following morning for my interview. The entire process was new to me. During my years with FAIR Autism Media, I had always been behind the camera, or the one asking questions — never in front of it. I was a little nervous and self-conscious. I tend to speak quickly when I'm passionate, and I worried my delivery might come across as too frenetic or that I'd overshare in my responses. But the producer conducting the interview, Gabe Rotello, was a seasoned professional who quickly helped put me at ease.

Our interview lasted ninety minutes. I had been provided a list of potential questions ahead of time, giving me the opportunity to reflect and prepare my responses. The night before, my brother Norman and I rehearsed them together. While my answers were still spontaneous and honest, they benefited from that preparation — I was more thoughtful in my word choices and more focused in how I told each story. This was before my memoir had surpassed 10,000 words, and much of what I shared hadn't yet been committed to paper. That interview became one of the first opportunities I had to articulate my experiences out loud, in sequence, with some degree of polish.

Afterward, both Gabe and another producer — who had been observing the interview from another room — approached me with praise. They were excited not just by how the interview went, but by the sheer depth and detail of my encounters. They also expressed genuine interest in the illustrations I had brought with me. I was asked to sign a media release giving Prometheus Entertainment permission to use the artwork in the episode — a request I was more than happy to accommodate.

Within days of returning to Chicago, I received a follow-up email from Gabe Rotello. As it turned out, the day after my interview, Gabe and his team had interviewed Whitley Strieber — author of *Communion*, and one of the most influential voices in abduction research. Gabe shared details of my case with Whitley, who expressed interest in connecting with me. Gabe then sent an email to both of us, facilitating the introduction.

Shortly after, Whitley and I spoke directly, and he invited me to appear on his Dreamland podcast — an offer I gladly accepted. After a few email exchanges, Mr. Strieber and I settled on recording an episode for his podcast on March 11th.

There was something symbolic about the sequence of events. First MUFON. Then Ancient Aliens. Then Whitley Strieber. It felt like stepping through layers—each more visible than the last. For years, I had lived in quiet reflection, alone with my memories. Now I was being given a microphone. Not just to share what happened to me, but to speak as one of them. One of the voices I used to listen to in search of clarity.

That realization didn't come without pressure. I knew the moment these episodes aired, there would be no going back. My name, my story, my face—out there. People would have opinions. Some would believe me. Others would dismiss me. But none of that could outweigh what this opportunity meant: for the first time, the truth of my experience would be heard without interruption.

It felt vulnerable, but also empowering. As if I had been handed back a part of myself that had been taken. Not my memories—those were still incomplete—but the ability to author the narrative. And as I prepared for my interview with Whitley, I began to sense that I was no longer just recounting the events. I was claiming them.

As exciting as the attention from MUFON and Ancient Aliens was, it didn't change the one thing I had come to expect from the phenomenon itself: silence. Nothing new had happened since March of 2024. And yet, the silence didn't feel final. It felt familiar. Measured. As though it, too, was part of a rhythm I hadn't fully recognized at first.

When I finally sat down for the Dreamland recording, there was a strange stillness in me. Not nerves. Not exactly excitement. Something more like gravity. Whitley's voice had been in my ears for years. I had listened to his books, watched his interviews, read his thoughts on contact, consciousness, and the soul. He had shaped the framework through which I first began to recognize my own experiences for what they were.

And now, here we were—face to face, even if only through a screen. He listened closely, asked thoughtful questions, and expressed astonishment at certain details of my story. More than once, he told me, "I've never heard anything quite like that." It wasn't flattery. It was recognition. And that meant everything.

To be seen in that way—by someone who had walked through his own fire, and emerged with language for the ineffable—was more affirming than I expected. I didn't feel like a guest on a podcast. I felt like someone crossing a threshold. From private experiencer to public witness. From isolation to conversation.

When the recording ended, I sat for a moment in silence. And I thought: maybe that's what we're all doing—those of us who choose to speak. We're not just telling stories. We're reclaiming the right to shape them.

And once I chose to speak, I knew I had to go further. Not just in sharing what happened—but in standing behind it. Publicly. Without ambiguity. That's what led me to take the next step.

15

THE MEASURE OF TRUTH

There comes a point in any extraordinary claim where belief alone is no longer enough—where conviction must be met with accountability. For me, that moment came in the spring of 2025, when I scheduled a polygraph examination to address the experiences detailed in this book. Not because I owed it to science, or skeptics, or even the media—but because I owed it to you, the reader.

The question was simple: could I prove that I'm telling the truth? The answer, of course, depends on what one considers proof. A polygraph is not a courtroom. It doesn't render verdicts. But it can reveal something deeper than hard evidence—it can measure consistency, certainty, and sincerity. It can test whether a person stands behind their own account without deception.

This was not a decision made lightly. I knew the risk. If I failed—if even one response showed deception—I'd be handing ammunition to every skeptic, every dismissive voice who ever called experiencers delusional, attention-seeking, or unstable. I knew what I was putting on the line. But I also knew something else: I've told the truth. And I'm not afraid to have that truth tested.

I began researching polygraph examiners in early April 2025. I didn't want a sensationalist or fringe operator—I wanted someone professional, experienced, and willing to take my case seriously. After reviewing several options, I settled on Central Polygraph Service in Northfield, Illinois. Their website was clean and direct, and their reputation solid. I sent an initial inquiry explaining that I had written a memoir about lifelong abduction experiences, and that I wanted to verify the truthfulness of key claims.

To their credit, they didn't flinch. Within a day or two, I received a reply from an examiner named Michael. We began exchanging emails about the nature of my request and, most importantly, the wording of the questions. That turned out to be trickier than expected. Polygraph questions need to be constructed with absolute clarity—no metaphors, no ambiguity, no emotionally loaded phrasing. After a few rounds of revision, we finalized two simple, direct questions:

1. Have you ever been physically present with a life form you considered to be a non-human alien?

2. Have you ever been physically touched by a life form you considered to be a non-human alien?

I paid for the session and scheduled the test for Wednesday, April 23rd, at 1:00 p.m. When the confirmation email arrived, I felt a strange blend of anticipation and pressure. I've done interviews. I've shared my story on camera. But this would be different. There's no rehearsal when electrodes are reading your pulse. No edits. No second takes. This time, the only thing that mattered was the truth—and how my body responded to it.

On the day of my test, I drove to Northfield, Illinois, an upscale suburb just north of Chicago. Central Polygraph's offices were located in a quiet office complex. After checking in, I was brought to a small exam room where Michael, the examiner, explained how the test would be conducted. The room was clinical and quiet. A computer desk, a few chairs against the wall, and a padded chair at the center with armrests and a pressure plate at the base. A wall-mounted camera faced the examinee, watching for subtle physical cues.

Michael walked me through the setup and connected the equipment: three finger sensors on my right hand, two straps across my chest, and my feet placed on the pressure plate. Once everything was in place, he began the baseline round. He instructed me to choose a number between 2 and 7. I chose 4. Then he asked me to deny having chosen each number—including 4—so the system could detect a known lie and use it as a control. My baseline readings were steady.

Then came the more personal questions. Some were meant to provoke an emotional response:

"Have you ever received sexual gratification as the result of interaction with a non-human alien?" That one caught me off guard. I thought, What the hell? But I answered "no," calmly, as instructed—no elaboration, no explanation.

Another pushed even harder: "Have you ever masturbated to pornography that was of a deviant or illegal nature?" I wanted to snap, Absolutely not, but again, I kept my voice level and said "no." These weren't accusations; they were stress tests, meant to trigger emotional response. And in my case, they didn't.

Then we reached the two relevant questions—the ones that truly mattered to me. "Have you ever been physically present with a life form you considered to be a non-human alien?"

"Yes," I answered, feeling the images flash across my memory: the garage encounter... the being on top of me in bed... the weight of presence that had never left me.

"Have you ever been physically touched by a life form you considered to be a non-human alien?"

"Yes," I said again, recalling the grey's hand in mine, the silent surgery, the hands on my abdomen. My heart didn't race—but my breath deepened.

That was my mistake.

The questions were repeated across four cycles. Each time, I remained still, my body controlled. But each time I reached those two questions, I unconsciously took deeper breaths. I didn't mean to. I wasn't afraid of the questions. But when I answered them, I felt them. I remembered. And that emotional charge—unintentional as it was—altered my physiology.

After the test, Michael disconnected the sensors and gestured toward the monitor, where my results were displayed in a chart of jagged lines and timestamps.

"Erik, your baseline is clean. Rock solid. You answered the control questions exactly as expected—flat and steady. But on the two relevant questions, you see this? You're totally calm when you say 'yes'—the white lines barely move—but then you take a deep breath right after. And the system reads that as a stress spike." He sighed and looked back at me.

"The software wants to fail you. But I've done this long enough to know that's not deception. That's emotion. I believe you were telling the truth. But because of those physiological spikes, I can't legally certify this result. I have to mark it as inconclusive."

In a strange way, the word 'inconclusive' felt all too familiar. It wasn't a verdict. It wasn't an accusation. It was a shrug. A non-answer that sounded like so many others I've heard across my life. When I've tried to tell someone about the encounters, the lights, the paralysis, the surgeries—I've been met with blank stares, polite nods, or awkward silence. Inconclusive. I've spent decades living in the grey space between belief and proof. And this result felt like just one more reminder that I don't fully belong in either world.

His words hit harder than I expected. I hadn't lied. But the test couldn't clear me. Not because of the content—but because of my humanity. Michael assured me I could retake the test—he was confident I would pass if I could regulate my breathing. But the cost of another session would set me back, and I'd need to wait. I left feeling both validated and disappointed. I hadn't failed. But I hadn't succeeded either.

Polygraphs have long played a curious, controversial role in the UFO and abduction landscape. For decades, they've been used by experiencers to lend credibility to stories that otherwise defy belief.

Take the case of Travis Walton, perhaps the most widely scrutinized abduction incident on record. In 1975, Walton vanished for five days in the Apache-Sitgreaves National Forest in Arizona. His logging crew—seven men in total—reported seeing him struck by a beam of light from a hovering craft. After his return, six of the witnesses took and passed polygraph tests administered by the Arizona Department of Public Safety, despite intense national attention and skepticism. Their results didn't prove what they saw—but they did prove they believed what they saw. That distinction matters. The tests became a cornerstone of the case's credibility, and for many of us since, a kind of rite of passage.

More than a decade earlier, Betty and Barney Hill had already walked that road. Their 1961 abduction experience in New Hampshire was the first to receive wide public attention in the United States. Under hypnosis, they independently recalled being taken aboard a craft, examined, and later returned. In the years that followed, they were interviewed by psychologists, scrutinized by the media, and eventually subjected to lie detector tests. Neither of them failed. While polygraph results from that era weren't handled with the rigor or documentation we expect today, their willingness to undergo such tests at all—at a time when interracial couples already faced prejudice—spoke volumes. They had nothing to gain. They simply wanted to be believed.

Skeptics, of course, are quick to point out the limitations. Polygraph results are generally inadmissible in court. The technology doesn't detect lies—it detects stress responses, physiological shifts that may (or may not) correlate with deception. False positives and false negatives can and do occur. Critics argue that a skilled liar can beat the machine, while a traumatized truth-teller can fail it. And they're right. The science is imperfect. But in the absence of medical proof, video documentation, or physical artifacts, the polygraph can still serve a powerful symbolic function. It shows a willingness to be examined. To face scrutiny. To put something sacred—your own memory—on the line.

For many abductees, taking a polygraph isn't about proving something to science. It's about reclaiming a small measure of agency. In a reality where control is often stripped from us—where we're taken without consent, returned without closure, and left to wrestle with fragments of memory—the decision to undergo a polygraph can feel like a defiant act of self-possession. We know the risks. We know the outcome might not favor us. And still, we go.

That's why I did it. Not because I believed it would silence every critic, or unlock every door, but because it felt like an honest gesture in a world where honesty is too easily dismissed. I didn't walk into that test expecting vindication. I walked in because I knew who I was. What had happened to me. And I wanted that certainty to meet the world in a visible, measurable way—even if the instrument wasn't perfect.

In the end, what does a polygraph really tell us? It tells us something about intention. About presence. It doesn't decode the mysteries of the phenomenon—but it offers a glimpse into how a person carries the weight of what they've seen. That matters. Especially when our stories are so often reduced to anecdote, myth, or pathology.

So yes, I'll likely take the test again. Not to prove the unprovable, but to show that I'm still standing in the center of my truth, unshaken. And if my breath hitches again—if memory overtakes biology—I'll face that, too.

Maybe that's the story. Maybe truth isn't always black and white on a graph. Maybe it can't be reduced to a spike or a dip in the lines.

I don't need a machine to know what happened to me. But I still want that clean pass. Not for validation—just for punctuation. To give this story a final, measurable beat.

In the end, though, maybe belief isn't measured in charts and wires at all. Maybe it's found in the willingness to step forward and say: this happened. I was there. And I'm not afraid to stand behind it. What I can offer is what I've offered from the start: my memory, my conviction, and my willingness to put it all on the line. And I do.

16

A CLOCKWORK GREY

History moves in circles, and in the grey space between memory and forgetting, the truth waits. As I look back on my experiences—and those of my mother—the frequency of visitations and the gaps between them suggest what could be a deliberate schedule the greys may follow with their abductees and their bloodlines.

As I've discussed earlier, my mother's encounters appeared to begin in 1953, though there's no telling if that was her first. Her next hint of visitation came in the early 1970s, when she began experiencing recurring nightmares of being chased by white orbs—the same orbs I saw while fully conscious between 1970 and 1974. It would seem my mother and I were both being visited during that four-year period, yet the key difference is that I have waking memories of the orbs, while she does not.

Then, twenty years later, in 1994, I had a waking memory of four small greys rushing out of my room in what I assume was an aborted abduction attempt. I also had impressions of what may have been visitations in 1995. If that's true, then 1994 wasn't an isolated event—it was likely part of another four-year cycle, during which I retained only one waking memory.

Then, twenty-five years after my last suspected visitation, the cycle began again. Between 2020 and 2024, I was taken every four to six weeks, on a schedule so regular that it became impossible to ignore.

Are these encounters indicative of a long-term, rotating schedule? If we assume that they visit every twenty years for four-year rotations of near-monthly abductions, what does that imply? What can we derive from this?

The Broader Phenomenon: Patterns in Visitation Schedules

If my own encounters followed a twenty-year cycle, with four-year periods of heightened activity, could this pattern extend beyond my case? Are other abductees experiencing similar visitations at structured intervals? A look at abduction research suggests that they are. While the frequency and timing of visitations vary between individuals, certain patterns have emerged across decades of testimony.

Some abductees report being taken on a near-monthly basis over an extended period. This kind of schedule aligns with what I experienced between 2020 and 2024, when visitations occurred roughly every four to six weeks. Whitley Strieber described periods where encounters happened in clusters, often recurring at predictable intervals in *Communion* and *Transformation*. He wrote about waking up to the presence of beings in his room repeatedly, sometimes as often as every few weeks, much like I experienced. Budd Hopkins, in *Intruders*, documented similar cases where abductees were taken regularly, especially those involved in reproductive experiments or hybrid integration efforts. David Jacobs found that those engaged in hybrid interactions were often taken every four to six weeks, a timeframe that exactly matches the frequency of my recent encounters. If the greys are engaged in long-term biological monitoring, whether through tissue collection, neurological scans, or tracking subtle physiological changes, then abductees may be subject to frequent check-ins to measure progress.

What's particularly unsettling about this short-term schedule is that it doesn't appear to be random. Instead, once an abductee enters an "active phase," they may be visited continuously for several years before the greys withdraw again. But why do they withdraw at all? If ongoing hybridization or genetic refinement is at the core of the abduction phenomenon, then these visitations likely have distinct phases—one period of intervention, then a long absence, perhaps to allow for adjustments to take effect.

A more disturbing pattern appears when looking at long-term tracking. Many abductees, like myself, report long gaps of twenty years or more before their experiences resume. Jim Sparks, in *The Keepers*, recalled an abduction pattern where he was taken repeatedly for a stretch of time, only to have decades of silence—until the cycle restarted. Similarly, cases in Barbara Lamb's regression work revealed abductees who realized they had been taken as children, then again decades later, often at key biological milestones. David Jacobs and Budd Hopkins both noted that abductees frequently reported their first experiences as children, then nothing for twenty or thirty years, until the cycle began again. This mirrors my own 1974, 1994, and 2020 pattern—three separate phases of abductions, each separated by roughly twenty years.

A Structured Agenda or Evolutionary Experiment?

If this twenty-year cycle is not unique to me but a common feature among abductees, then we must ask: What purpose does this timing serve? The idea that the greys return at such precise intervals suggests something deeply methodical, whether it is a pre-determined schedule of genetic harvesting, a long-term observational study, or a gradual acclimation process for abductees.

One possible reason for these cycles is that the greys are tracking something specific within the abductees they repeatedly take—perhaps a biological or neurological marker that only becomes relevant at certain stages of life. If their primary goal involves tissue collection, reproductive intervention, or hybridization efforts, then it would make sense that they return at key biological milestones. The greys may not need constant surveillance but rather periodic re-engagement when their subjects reach the next phase of development—whether that development occurs naturally or as a result of prior abductions.

This could explain why each round of visitations appears different from the last. In my earlier encounters, their interest seemed primarily focused on reproductive extraction, yet later, their interactions shifted toward tissue samples, surgical interventions, and potentially even neurological mapping. It's as if they are following an internal roadmap, fine-tuning something over time, rather than simply repeating the same procedures with every cycle.

If hybridization is their focus, then each twenty-year interval could represent the time required for a new hybrid generation to reach maturity before abductees are taken again to contribute fresh genetic material for another round. This would imply that abductees are not just subjects of study but active genetic resources, drawn into a system that repeats across multiple human lifetimes.

The Psychological Component: Conditioning Over Time

The cycle may not be driven by biology alone. If the greys have mastered neurological manipulation, it's possible they space out their encounters intentionally to shape abductees' perceptions, behaviors, and cognitive processes in a controlled manner.

Four years of intense experiences is long enough to create lasting memories but short enough that abductees do not become fully accustomed to their presence. Then, by withdrawing for twenty years, they ensure that abductees age, mature, and enter new life stages, changing their perspectives before they are re-engaged. This could serve a dual purpose: allowing them to assess the long-term effects of their interventions, while also making sure abductees mentally reset, suppress, or reinterpret their experiences over time.

If their goal is to acclimate abductees gradually to their presence, then these long absences may not be pauses at all—but rather, calculated periods of psychological reshaping before the next stage begins.

The gaps allow abductees to normalize their past encounters, which may, in turn, alter their receptiveness when the greys return.

Tracking Generations, Not Just Individuals

This leads to an even more unsettling possibility. If my mother's experiences in 1953 preceded my own starting in 1970, then this pattern may not just be about individuals, but rather entire bloodlines. The idea that the greys are following specific family lines is well-documented in abduction research, with cases of multi-generational contact occurring across decades.

Budd Hopkins and David Jacobs both explored cases in which abductees realized that their own children were also being taken—sometimes at the same ages they themselves had been. Often, parents only suspect this after noticing strange behaviors in their children, such as unexplained fears, sleep disturbances, or oddly specific dreams that seem far too detailed for a child's imagination. Some abductees have even recalled waking up to see their children missing from their beds—only to reappear later as if nothing had happened.

I have no definitive proof that my daughter was ever taken, but there was one experience that has never sat right with me. After one of my own abductions, when I found myself back in my bed, I lay there in the darkness, my body heavy with that familiar post-encounter fatigue. Then, through our shared wall, I heard laughter. It was Miranda.

She was 23 years old at the time, but due to her nonverbal autism, she has the mind of a child. Hearing her awake in the middle of the night wasn't unheard of, but something about this moment felt different.

She wasn't just laughing—she was giggling, entertained, as though someone had been playing with her. A slow unease crept over me. I listened, waiting for another sound—movement, the creak of her bed, anything to indicate that she was merely stirring from a dream. But the house was otherwise silent.

Who had made her laugh?

Of course, I can't prove she experienced anything that night. Maybe she was dreaming. Maybe there was nothing unusual about it.

But I couldn't shake the feeling that, while the Greys had just left me, they hadn't left the house.

If abductions truly follow bloodlines, then it stands to reason that they are not only tracking genetic markers but also observing how abductees' children respond to contact. Some researchers believe this may be a form of acclimation, where young abductees are introduced gradually so that they do not develop the same level of fear that older generations experience.

If true, this raises a disturbing question: Are some abductees' children being conditioned to accept the Greys from an early age? Could that explain why Miranda awoke laughing?

I can only speculate. But if history repeats itself, as it has with my mother and me, then I may not be the last in my family to experience these encounters.

A Process That Never Ends

When I take a step back and look at the pattern, it becomes clear that this is not an isolated phenomenon. The recurring cycles, the multi-generational involvement, and the gradual changes in focus across different phases of abduction all suggest something deliberate and ongoing.

The nature of this process raises an even more unsettling question: To what end?

If the greys have been conducting these abductions for decades—possibly centuries—then what exactly is the final objective? Are they simply testing and refining their hybridization methods, adjusting variables each cycle? Or is this process building toward a larger goal—one that is still beyond our understanding?

If this cycle truly never ends, then abductees like myself are part of something far bigger than we realize. What's unclear is whether we are merely biological resources being used to further their agenda, or if we are being shaped into something else entirely.

Some abductees have reported changes over time—not just physically, but mentally. The longer the encounters persist, the more they notice subtle alterations in their thoughts, emotions, and perceptions. Could prolonged exposure to the greys be rewiring abductees in ways that aren't immediately obvious? And if so, to what purpose?

If their interactions with us are meant to be cumulative, then abductees are not simply test subjects in a repeating experiment—we may be part of an unfolding process, one that will continue for generations until they achieve their endgame.

Whatever that may be. I'll speculate on this, later.

The Spaces Between: What Happens During the Silent 20-Year Gaps?

If the greys operate on a structured timeline, withdrawing for two decades before re-engaging, then the natural question is: Do they truly disappear during those years, or are they simply watching from a distance? The absence of direct encounters does not necessarily mean that abductees are free from their influence.

While I never had forewarnings of their return, I do not believe that their twenty-year absences are complete disengagements. Rather, I suspect that the greys have the ability to monitor abductees continuously, even during the so-called silent years. My encounters suggest that they know exactly where I am, what condition I am in, and when to return.

Many abductees report feeling watched in periods between encounters, yet the evidence suggests that their surveillance is more than just psychological. The idea that the greys can track their subjects remotely is not new. Numerous accounts describe abductees receiving implants—small, metallic objects embedded deep in soft tissue, often in places difficult to detect or remove. These objects, sometimes discovered in nasal cavities, ears, or limbs, have been suspected of serving as biological tracking devices.

If the greys are using such devices, it would explain how they are able to locate abductees immediately upon their return cycle. It would also suggest that their twenty-year gaps are not gaps at all—only a period where their interaction shifts from direct involvement to passive observation. If they have implanted tracking devices, it's likely that these are capable of not just pinpointing an abductee's location, but also transmitting data on their health, neurological state, and genetic composition.

There is also the possibility that they do not need physical devices at all. If the greys possess an advanced understanding of electromagnetic fields, bio-signatures, or quantum entanglement, they may have the ability to remotely monitor abductees through means we do not yet understand. The notion of telepathic surveillance has been raised in abductee reports, with some claiming to have experienced random moments of mental "intrusion" during off-periods, as if something external had briefly tapped into their thoughts.

Even if direct telepathic surveillance is not occurring, there is reason to believe that abductees may still be subtly influenced or primed for the next wave. Some researchers have speculated that abductees undergo periods of neurological preparation—a kind of long-term conditioning process that ensures that when the cycle resumes, the abductee will be more compliant, more receptive, or more neurologically optimized for whatever procedure or extraction is required next.

For the greys, time may not function the way it does for us. The twenty-year interval could be an instant from their perspective—a controlled pause before the next stage of their operation. If their methods of observation are so advanced that they can gather everything they need without direct abduction, then the moments we perceive as "gaps" in their presence may be nothing more than a shift in operational focus.

If the pattern holds true, then what they do in these silent years is just as important as what they do during their active years.

Whether the twenty-year gap is dictated by the maturation of hybrids, the accumulation of genetic adaptations, or the psychological management of abductees, one thing is certain:

Even when they are gone, they are not really gone.

The twenty-year gap does not erase the past. It lingers in the mind, an ever-present question: When will they return? You go about your life, convincing yourself that maybe—just maybe—it's over. But the unease never fully fades. Every unexplainable dream, every shadow in the corner of your vision, every odd sensation of being watched—it all fuels the question: Are they still there?

If the pattern holds true, then what they do in these silent years is just as important as what they do during their active years.

A Cycle Without an End—or a Final Phase?

If the greys operate on a structured schedule, returning for abductees every twenty years, then it raises a deeper question: Does the cycle ever end? Or does an abductee remain useful to them for life—perhaps even beyond?

Many abductees assume that their encounters are temporary, that they are part of an experiment that will eventually conclude. But my experiences suggest otherwise. Each return cycle has been different, yet it has never truly stopped. I have never received any indication that the greys intend to "release" me from their program. The more I study these patterns, the more I wonder: Is there a final stage? Do abductees ever become obsolete to them?

It would be easy to assume that abductees are useful only as long as they are reproductively viable—that once sperm or egg quality declines, their role in the program would end. But evidence from other lifelong abductees contradicts this assumption. Many abductees report being taken well into old age, sometimes into their seventies or eighties, long past their reproductive years. This suggests that the greys are not just interested in sperm or eggs—they are collecting something more enduring, something that remains valuable for an entire lifetime.

One possible explanation is that even when reproductive viability ends, an abductee's genetic material is still useful in other ways. If the greys are harvesting DNA not just for hybridization but for biological engineering, then even aging abductees could provide stem cells, epigenetic data, and neurological mapping.

Research into stem cell potential supports this idea. Even after reproductive decline, bone marrow remains a rich source of hematopoietic stem cells, which are known to regenerate blood, immune cells, and even certain tissues (*Goodell et al.*, 2015). If the greys are refining their hybrid genetics over multiple human generations, bone marrow may provide the stable genetic material they need, even after reproductive usefulness has passed. The use of stem cells in regenerative medicine is a major field of human research (*Trounson & McDonald*, 2015), and it's reasonable to speculate that the greys, with their superior biological knowledge, would be utilizing similar processes—perhaps at a level beyond our understanding.

Beyond genetics, the greys may also have an interest in neurological tracking. Many abductees have reported undergoing procedures that involve headgear, brain scans, or even what appears to be memory extraction (*Hopkins*, 1987; *Jacobs*, 1998). If their interest extends beyond genetics and into consciousness itself, then abductees may be useful even in later life stages as their minds and cognitive abilities change. Studies on aging and neural plasticity show that the brain continues to adapt and rewire itself throughout life (*Pascual-Leone et al.*, 2005), which could explain why the greys continue monitoring abductees well beyond their reproductive years. They may be observing how neural pathways shift over decades—perhaps even measuring the long-term effects of repeated abductions on human cognition.

There is also the question of epigenetic tracking. While DNA remains stable throughout a person's life, epigenetic markers change, influenced by environment, aging, stress, and even external manipulation (*Jaenisch & Bird*, 2003). If the greys are monitoring how genetic modifications made in earlier abductions manifest in later life stages, they may need to return to abductees periodically to assess the long-term results of their work. Scientists have already begun to explore how epigenetic inheritance may affect future generations (*Jirtle &*

Skinner, 2007), which could indicate that the greys are not just monitoring one generation, but entire genetic lineages over time.

All of this suggests that abductees do not "age out" of the program. Even if the focus shifts over time, abductees remain useful to the greys at every stage of life.

If the twenty-year cycle holds, then my next phase should occur in 2040. If I am still alive, what will they need from me at that point? If they were previously focused on reproductive material, will they now shift their focus to neurological function, cognitive shifts, or stem cell harvesting? Or will the process simply continue indefinitely, cycling abductees through different phases of usefulness until the end of their natural life?

There is even a more unsettling possibility—that an abductee's usefulness does not end at death. Some abductees have reported memories of being taken to clinical, morgue-like environments, where they saw deceased humans being examined (*Strieber*, 1987; *Jacobs*, 2015). If the greys' program is truly longitudinal, spanning entire lifetimes, then it may not stop simply because the body dies. Are they still collecting data post-mortem? Are they harvesting genetic material from the deceased?

If abductees do not age out of the program, then the final phase may not be retirement—but something else entirely.

17

INSIDE THE TRANCE

"We are such stuff as dreams are made on, and our little life is rounded with a sleep."
— William Shakespeare, *The Tempest*

There is a kind of sleep that is not rest. A state where the body is present but the self is adrift — not dreaming, not awake, but suspended in something else entirely. I have been placed in that state more times than I can count. Inside the trance, time loses meaning. So does fear. It is not peace, but stillness. And in that stillness, I am no longer a person to them — just a tool to be used, unresisting and silent.

Throughout this book, I've shared many of the strange and deeply personal experiences I've had with the beings commonly referred to as the Greys. In nearly every encounter, one detail repeats with chilling consistency: I am entranced. My body becomes paralyzed. My emotions are dulled to the point of nonexistence. Physical sensations are muted or absent. I am wide awake but reduced to a passive observer, unable to act, speak, or even feel alarmed.

This altered state is one of the most overlooked and least understood aspects of the abduction phenomenon. And yet, it may be one of the most revealing. What does it mean to have your consciousness manipulated so precisely — not knocked out, but held in place? What kind of force or intelligence can bypass the body's survival instincts so seamlessly? And perhaps most disturbing: how close are we, as a species, to replicating this kind of control ourselves?

In this chapter, I'd like to explore that state of entrancement in greater depth — not just as I experienced it, but as it relates to what we know from psychology, medicine, and neuroscience. From clinical paralysis to emotional suppression, from hypnotic trance to military experiments in mind control, I believe the nature of this silent, imposed stillness deserves careful attention.

To ground this exploration, I'll return briefly to a moment I've already shared — one that occurred in 2020, inside my own garage.

When I became conscious, I was suspended off my feet and staring down at a small grey, illuminated on one side by a light that streamed through the garage window. I felt almost nothing, both physically and emotionally. It was as if my only working sense was my eyes. While mostly naked, I could hardly feel the cold air of the April night upon my skin. Anything below my neck was paralyzed. More surprising was my emotional state. My fear response was gone. My heart rate didn't increase, the hairs on my extremities didn't stand on end. I felt no panic. When the grey "spoke" to me using telepathy, I had receptive language... I understood the message. But I couldn't PONDER the words. I couldn't even think of a question or response. My brain's ability to express was as muted as my entire nervous system. This experience would become a common theme in my relationship with the Greys.

Parallels in Science and Medicine

What I experienced in that garage — and in many other encounters — has elements that defy easy classification. But over time, I began to notice that certain aspects of the trance state share features with conditions recognized in sleep research, neuropsychology, and even anesthesia. None are a perfect fit. But the overlaps are revealing.

Sleep Paralysis: The Misfit Explanation

Sleep paralysis is often the go-to explanation used by skeptics to dismiss abduction accounts. It involves a temporary inability to move or speak while falling asleep or waking up, often accompanied by hallucinations or the vivid sense of a presence in the room. It can be terrifying — the mind is alert, but the body remains locked in the stillness of REM atonia. Some people report shadowy figures, a crushing weight on the chest, or an overwhelming feeling of evil. It's understandable why this explanation is applied to abduction accounts.

According to a 2011 review published in *Sleep Medicine Reviews*, isolated sleep paralysis occurs in about 7.6% of the general population, with higher rates among people with PTSD or sleep disruptions. The condition is characterized by REM intrusion, where muscle atonia continues briefly into waking consciousness. A related phenomenon, hypnopompic hallucination — vivid imagery experienced while waking from sleep — occurs in roughly 12% of the population and is often grouped into the same category.

These events can produce disorienting visions, feelings of presence, or even physical sensations — but they are generally brief, fragmented, and accompanied by the clear sense that one is waking from something. In contrast, my experiences were marked not by emergence from sleep, but by sudden, externally imposed immobilization while already awake — a shift into a state of calm paralysis with no dream logic or drowsiness. They weren't internalized hallucinations. They were observed invasions.

Anthropologist David J. Hufford, in his landmark book *The Terror That Comes in the Night,* documented cross-cultural accounts of what he called the "Old Hag" phenomenon — sleep paralysis combined with hallucinated assaults by entities. Hufford was one of the first to suggest that not all sleep paralysis fits neatly into a psychological box, and that some cases may reflect actual anomalous experiences, possibly even involving non-human intelligences. He referred to this as "the experiential source hypothesis."

I've never experienced true sleep paralysis in the traditional medical sense — only something close to it during my 1994 encounter with the four greys. That morning, I awoke to find myself paralyzed, overwhelmed by panic, and fought with everything I had to break free. Somehow, I did. The greys seemed startled by my resistance and left the room in a hurry. It was nothing like the trance states I experienced during later abductions. Those were eerily calm. There was no panic, no thrashing against my body — only a still, sterile obedience that felt foreign to who I am. That absence of fear — that emotionally deadened compliance — is precisely what makes the trance states so difficult to explain.

Whitley Strieber addresses this distinction in *Communion*, noting that while his body was often immobilized during encounters, the experience never aligned with any dream-state paralysis. "Sleep paralysis," he wrote, "is characterized by the immediate return of control. This was not like that. This was a taking." The clarity of his awareness, the presence of non-human beings, and the aftereffects all pointed to something more structured, more invasive.

Budd Hopkins, too, rejected the sleep paralysis model. In *Missing Time* and *Intruders*, he documented case after case in which the paralysis occurred during waking hours — while driving, standing, or walking. These were not sleep transitions. The affected individuals were pulled into the trance-like state mid-activity, often in full daylight. The pattern was too consistent — and too surgically precise — to be explained by dream-state carryover.

Dr. David Jacobs, in *The Threat*, went further. He noted that sleep paralysis typically ends in seconds or minutes. But abductees often report extended missing time, lasting 30 minutes to several hours, along with marks on the body, unusual fatigue, or implanted memories that surface under hypnosis. He argued that the sleep paralysis explanation was a convenient defense mechanism for both experiencers and investigators — a way to dismiss what the conscious mind struggles to integrate.

If the garage experience had simply been sleep paralysis, I would have been frozen in my bed. But I wasn't in bed. I was awake, upright, and not inside my house. What followed was not the chaotic panic of a nightmare, but the muted quiet of something else entirely. This wasn't the "Old Hag" pressing down on my chest. It was a highly controlled encounter with a being that didn't need to frighten me — because it had already removed the part of me that could be frightened.

Dissociation and Emotional Detachment

In the psychological field, dissociation is a state in which a person becomes detached from their thoughts, feelings, body, or surroundings. According to the *Diagnostic and Statistical Manual of Mental Disorders (DSM-5)*, dissociative disorders involve a *"disruption or discontinuity in the normal integration of consciousness, memory, identity, emotion, perception, body representation, motor control, and behavior."* It's most common among trauma survivors, particularly those who have experienced chronic abuse, sexual violence, or severe stress.

Dissociation serves as a kind of psychological escape hatch — the mind distancing itself from the present to protect against unbearable stimuli. In extreme cases, this includes depersonalization (a feeling of being detached from oneself) and derealization (a sense that the world around you is unreal or distorted). Psychiatrist Daphne Simeon, who co-authored *Feeling Unreal*, writes that depersonalization can feel like *"being a spectator to one's own life, as if watching a movie."*

That's where this begins to intersect with the abduction experience. The feeling of being emotionally numb, of observing passively from somewhere behind your own eyes, is familiar to those who have endured both dissociation and the trance state imposed during abductions. But the difference is critical: dissociation is internally driven — a coping response generated by the psyche. What I experienced felt externally imposed — as if something had reached in and switched off my emotional circuitry.

As trauma expert Bessel van der Kolk notes in *The Body Keeps the Score*, trauma survivors often *"disconnect from their emotions in order to survive,*" and in doing so, their bodies remain physically present while their emotional experience is suppressed. But my emotional flattening didn't come from within. I wasn't responding to overwhelming fear. There was no fear to begin with. The numbness wasn't a defense — it was a condition delivered to me.

This distinction matters. Abduction accounts often describe experiencers being fully conscious yet eerily passive — watching procedures unfold, seeing beings move around them, and yet remaining emotionally inert. David Jacobs has described this repeatedly in his hypnosis work, noting that abductees often recall their experiences with a shocking lack of emotion — not because they're repressing trauma, but because something removed their capacity to feel in the moment.

In one case recounted in *Walking Among Us*, an abductee described being awake on a table, surrounded by beings performing a procedure, but said she felt nothing — not even curiosity. When asked why she didn't scream or move, she replied, "It didn't occur to me to try." That kind of cognitive quieting — a complete shutdown of will — is not something trauma alone can explain.

There was no panic to shut down. No mounting terror to escape. My emotional flattening didn't come from psychological protection — it came from manipulation, from an outside force that had no need to traumatize me when it could simply remove my ability to feel.

Anesthesia Awareness: Conscious but Frozen

A lesser-known but well-documented medical phenomenon is anesthesia awareness — when a patient remains conscious during surgery but is unable to move or signal distress. Though paralyzed by muscle relaxants, their brain remains awake, sometimes even capable of feeling pain. In some cases, patients recall floating sensations. Others hear snippets of conversation from the surgical team. And many describe it as a kind of living nightmare — not because of the pain, but because of the helplessness. No matter how intensely they try to scream or move, nothing happens.

According to a study published in *Anesthesiology* (Ghoneim & Block, 1997), intraoperative awareness occurs in approximately 1–2 out of every 1,000 patients receiving general anesthesia. Though rare, the psychological impact can be lasting. Some develop symptoms of PTSD. Others refuse further surgeries altogether.

One of the most well-known cases is Carol Weihrer, a patient who awoke during eye surgery and later testified before Congress. "I was awake," she said. "I felt every cut. I heard everything. I was paralyzed. And nobody knew." Her case became a cornerstone of patient rights advocacy in the early 2000s.

That's the closest medical parallel I've found to the trance state I experienced. But in my case, there was no hospital. No surgical team. No anesthesia cocktail. I was awake, aware, paralyzed — and emotionally muted. The numbness wasn't a medical error. It wasn't a failure of sedation. It felt like an engineered state. A precise configuration of awareness that had been dialed in for a purpose.

I've also undergone medical sedation — a colonoscopy under propofol, for instance — and I remember how quickly unconsciousness set in after the drug entered my bloodstream. I couldn't hear people talking, but I could hear the beeping of equipment throughout the procedure. Even under heavy sedation, some sensory input leaked through. But it was murky, dreamlike. There was no lucidity. No presence. And when I woke up, I felt groggy, displaced. It was a clean medical experience, but nothing like what I experienced with the Greys. Their version of paralysis wasn't fogged by chemicals. It was crystal clear, and that's what makes it so chilling. I wasn't sedated. I was taken offline.

Whitley Strieber, in *Transformation*, described being subjected to procedures while conscious, yet strangely unafraid. "I didn't feel like a victim," he wrote. "I didn't feel much of anything. I watched what was being done to me, and it was... clinical." That word has stayed with me. Clinical. Detached. As though the beings involved had not only suppressed pain, but had disabled the emotional mechanisms that make an experience feel human.

I've never forgotten that sense of being frozen while something watched me. And I've often wondered if that state — stripped of pain, stripped of resistance, yet filled with presence — is exactly what they want. Not an unconscious body. Not a sedated mind. But a neutralized witness.

Hypnosis: Willing Trance, Unwilling Subject

Hypnosis is perhaps the most fascinating parallel — and the most unsettling. Under hypnosis, a subject enters a focused, suggestible state in which memories can be retrieved, perceptions altered, and even pain blocked. The subject may not remember things said or done under hypnosis, or may recall vivid past experiences long thought forgotten. But hypnosis, as it's understood in therapy or entertainment, requires a degree of cooperation. The subject must willingly enter the trance state — and can usually leave it just as willingly.

According to Dr. David Spiegel, a psychiatrist and hypnosis researcher at Stanford University, hypnosis involves "a shift in brain activity that reduces the influence of executive control systems," particularly in the dorsolateral prefrontal cortex — the part of the brain associated with self-reflection and critical evaluation. In brain imaging studies, Spiegel found that hypnotized individuals experience reduced connectivity between this executive center and the salience network, which monitors external stimuli. In simpler terms, the brain stops questioning and becomes more receptive to suggestion.

But it's still a collaborative act. Hypnosis only works when the subject allows it — when they choose to lower the gates of control. That's the critical difference.

What I experienced bore a strange resemblance to hypnosis — but without consent. My body was immobilized, my attention narrowed, and my memory became hazy or fragmented. It was a trance, yes — but one enforced by something far more precise than suggestion. I wasn't led into the state by voice or rhythm. There was no countdown, no command. One moment I was present, and the next, I was held — as if something far beyond our understanding of hypnosis had reached inside and toggled the necessary switches.

Milton Erickson, considered the father of modern hypnotherapy, believed hypnosis was "a special psychological state with certain physiological attributes, resembling sleep only superficially and marked by a functioning of the individual at a level of awareness other than the ordinary conscious state." I agree — but what I experienced wasn't an alternate state of my choosing. It was imposed upon me. Not induced. Not invited. Enforced.

In one sense, it was like hypnosis — but perfected. Not a practice. A technology. Not a guided trance, but a neural override. There were no visible tools, no external stimuli I could detect. And yet, my emotional spectrum collapsed, my thoughts flattened, my will evaporated. It wasn't suggestibility. It was compliance, built into the structure of the moment.

It was as if the Greys had refined the mechanism of trance far beyond what we've achieved. Not a psychological trick, but a consciousness bypass. Hypnosis, but weaponized.

The Emotional Silence

Of all the elements that make up the trance state, the most difficult to explain — and the hardest to live with — is the absence of fear. During my encounters, even in moments where I was confronted with the unknown, even when I was physically vulnerable or surrounded by non-human entities, there was no rising panic. No dread. No instinctive response that should have triggered a scream or a struggle.

Instead, there was a kind of emotional vacuum — a stillness so complete it felt inhuman. I didn't resist because I couldn't. Not due to physical restraints, but because the will to resist had been taken offline. That's not something most people can imagine unless they've experienced it themselves. It's not numbness born of shock — it's numbness born of design.

In psychiatry, a condition known as *flat affect* is used to describe patients who show little or no emotion, often due to brain injury or disorders like schizophrenia. But even those cases come with disorientation or dysfunction. What I experienced was coldly functional — my ability to feel had been surgically silenced, yet my awareness remained sharp.

This emotional silence was often accompanied by a clarity of observation. I could see and remember details. I was mentally present — just not emotionally. It's as though they turned off only what they needed to in order to make me manageable: panic, anger, defiance. The rest was left intact so I could comply, observe, and perhaps even process what they wanted me to witness.

David Jacobs has written extensively about this in *Walking Among Us*, noting that many abductees describe their experiences in a strikingly flat, almost indifferent tone. He believes this is not repression, but the result of an imposed mental state. In one case, a woman described being surrounded by beings while something was inserted into her body — and her only emotional response at the time was curiosity. Not fear. Not embarrassment. Just a quiet, muted intrigue.

Whitley Strieber, too, has reflected on the calmness he felt in situations that would normally trigger terror. He described it as "a quieting of the soul," a soft suppression of instinct so complete that he sometimes questioned if he had done it to himself — or if they had done it to him.

What does that say about them? About their knowledge of our biology, our neurology? If they can suppress fear without shutting down consciousness, they understand us at a level far beyond anything we can replicate. It also raises an unsettling possibility: what if they want us aware — just not resistant? What if the goal isn't to render us unconscious, but to let us see and remember just enough, without giving us the emotional tools to fight back?

The silence they impose isn't mercy. It's control. And in some ways, it's the most invasive violation of all — not the stealing of a body, but the quiet erasure of selfhood, one feeling at a time.

The Implication of Control

The trance state, in all its variations, points to one unavoidable conclusion: control is the point. Not just control over movement, but over emotion, perception, and will. The Greys don't merely immobilize — they disarm, neurologically and psychologically. And they do it without restraint, without sedation, without struggle. That's the most revealing part.

There's something surgical about the way they do it. As if they know exactly which cognitive switches need to be flipped to render a human docile — not asleep, not drugged, but quiet. It suggests not just a familiarity with human neurology, but a working mastery of it. They know what to suppress. They know how to isolate consciousness from emotion, and how to mute the fight-or-flight response without muting awareness itself.

In 1969, the RAND Corporation published a document titled *UFOs: What to Do?*, speculating on the psychological implications of contact scenarios. Though dry and couched in academic language, the authors acknowledged the possibility that "control over perception and behavior" could be a defining aspect of a non-human intelligence's interaction with humans. It was a rare moment of institutional candor — and it aligns uncomfortably well with what abductees have reported for decades.

David Jacobs has pointed out that the Greys rarely waste effort on restraint or sedation because they don't need to. Once the subject is entranced, resistance is gone. The desire to resist is gone. It's not just paralysis — it's a pre-programmed mental compliance. And that implies a far more intimate understanding of us than most people are ready to consider.

What's more disturbing is that they don't need to convince, or even coerce. Once the trance begins, compliance is automatic. There's no inner monologue screaming for freedom. There's no moral conflict or mental protest. They don't just paralyze the body. They erase the impulse to object. In that sense, the trance state isn't just a tool of abduction — it's a method of dominion. A kind of nonviolent possession.

Strieber, in *The Key*, speculated that the visitors had learned to interface with the human nervous system directly — not through machines, but through consciousness itself. He asked the question: What if they don't use tools because they are the tool? That idea has haunted me. The notion that the beings themselves — or their minds — may be the mechanism of control. That there's no gap between will and effect. That they simply decide, and it happens.

And it works. I was there. I watched it happen from within my own body, and I did nothing. Not because I lacked courage — but because I lacked permission to be myself. That permission had been quietly revoked. My mind was not asleep. It had been seized — softly, clinically, and completely.

Returning from the Trance

Coming out of the trance state isn't something I've ever done on my own. I don't gradually recover sensation or emotion. There's no tingling in the limbs, no slow surfacing of awareness like waking from sleep. Instead, the transition is instant and absolute — because I'm not the one making it.

I'm conscious when they need me to be, and unconscious when they're finished. That's the pattern. There's no in-between state, no control on my end. One moment I'm there, fully paralyzed but observing. The next, I wake up back home with no memory of how I got there — just the haunting certainty that I was somewhere else, being used for something I didn't understand.

Budd Hopkins, in *Witnessed*, described several cases in which abductees "woke up" in unfamiliar locations before being returned to bed, with no recollection of the transport. Many remembered only two slivers of awareness: the moment they were taken, and the moment they were dropped back. The rest was a void.

For me, the emotional delay was often just as striking. There were encounters I came out of feeling nothing at all — not even fear. It was as though the emotional volume had been turned to zero and never fully restored. In some cases, it took hours or even days before I felt real again — before I could grieve what I'd just gone through, or even name it.

That delay raises uncomfortable questions: what else was delayed? Were memories still forming and then being erased? Was perception only partially restored? What if the real damage — or the most profound contact — occurred during the gaps? The places I wasn't allowed to keep?

David Jacobs has emphasized this same pattern in his regression work — the sense that some memories are deliberately excluded from conscious access. Not blocked by trauma, but scrubbed clean by the phenomenon itself. In some cases, he said, the memories "feel missing in real time," as if the experiencer is watching their own perception being shaped and pruned like film on an editing reel.

The return doesn't feel like waking. It feels like being returned. Like something borrowed me — consciousness, body, identity — and gave me back only when it was done. And I often wonder: Did I come back whole? Or was some part of me left behind, still paused in that place of silence, still watching, still held?

Replicating the Trance

If we set aside the question of who or what is behind the abduction phenomenon and look purely at the mechanics of the trance state, one question becomes unavoidable: could we replicate it? Could modern science — or some clandestine subset of it — induce the same kind of full-body paralysis, emotional suppression, and carefully tuned consciousness that I've experienced in the presence of the Greys?

On the surface, it seems unlikely. And yet, when you examine the current state of neuroscience, pharmacology, and mind control research, the question becomes more uncomfortable. Because the answer is: not exactly... but we are alarmingly close.

In clinical settings, we already possess tools to immobilize the human body without affecting consciousness. Neuromuscular blockers such as succinylcholine are widely used during surgeries to paralyze skeletal muscles, preventing movement even if the patient remains aware. If administered without proper sedation — whether accidentally or through negligence — the result is a fully conscious, completely paralyzed human being, locked inside themselves, unable to scream, gesture, or escape. It's considered a rare but devastating form of anesthesia failure. And yet, the condition exists. We have already touched this edge of control, however unintentionally.

More recently, non-invasive techniques such as **Transcranial Magnetic Stimulation (TMS)** have shown that it's possible to interfere directly with brain activity through magnetic pulses. By targeting specific areas of the motor cortex, researchers have been able to disable voluntary movement in a subject's limbs — essentially flipping off sections of agency while leaving consciousness untouched. The applications for treating depression and neurological disorders are promising. But behind those promises lies a deeper implication: if we can interrupt movement remotely with precision, how far are we from suppressing intention itself?

In the emotional domain, we already wield pharmacological tools capable of muting the body's survival instincts. Drugs like ketamine dissociate emotion from perception, allowing a person to observe trauma with a sense of detachment. Under its influence, pain and fear become abstractions — intellectual events devoid of visceral consequence. Midazolam, a benzodiazepine, is used in hospitals and interrogation rooms alike for its ability to cause anterograde amnesia — meaning subjects can follow commands and carry out tasks they'll never remember. And propranolol, a beta-blocker, has been shown to blunt the physiological effects of terror by reducing heart rate and adrenaline response, effectively silencing the body's scream before it begins.

Combine these effects — dissociation, amnesia, emotional dulling — and you have something very close to the Greys' method of control. But still, these are brute-force tools. They work by flooding the system, not by targeting specific circuits. The trance state I experienced didn't feel drugged or altered. It felt designed. It was silent, clean, and surgically specific. It allowed my mind to observe while stripping away only what was inconvenient — emotion, resistance, identity. The rest remained perfectly functional.

There is also the matter of frequency-based influence — a topic that once lived solely on the fringes of science, but is now part of mainstream exploration. Binaural beats, auditory illusions created by playing slightly different tones in each ear, have been shown to influence brainwave states. Theta waves, associated with trance and deep meditation, can be induced by manipulating sound frequency. Meanwhile, pulsed electromagnetic fields have been tested for their ability to alter mood, sleep cycles, and even short-term cognition. These are not theories — they are published experiments, many conducted under the umbrella of non-lethal defense technology.

During the Cold War, both the United States and the Soviet Union devoted significant resources to the possibility of mind manipulation. The now-infamous MK-Ultra program explored the use of LSD, sensory deprivation, isolation, hypnosis, and trauma as tools for behavior control. Though the program's records were largely destroyed, what remains reveals a chilling ambition: the creation of a human subject who could be observed, altered, or erased — with or without their awareness. The legacy of MK-Ultra is not just conspiracy fodder. It is evidence that the question of consciousness control has already been asked — and that the people asking it were not science fiction authors, but government psychologists.

To replicate the trance state I encountered would require a fusion of technologies and techniques — the ability to override motor function remotely, to suppress emotional reactivity without sedation, to selectively block memory while preserving lucid awareness. And perhaps most disturbingly, to return the subject to normalcy with no external trace. No scars. No sedation hangover. No flinching when the lights come on.

The experience didn't feel like the result of experimentation. It felt like the product of mastery. The Greys know how we work — neurologically, psychologically, spiritually. They don't merely control us physically. They isolate and disengage the mechanisms that make us "us." They bypass the human soul's defenses as if it were an outdated firewall. They don't need wires, restraints, or drugs. They don't even need verbal commands. Their method of control appears to be something far more intimate — something that speaks directly to the interface between consciousness and biology.

That's what makes it so chilling. Because what they achieve — silencing a person's agency while leaving their eyes open and their mind intact — is not some mystical impossibility. It's a technology. Perhaps biological, perhaps electromagnetic, perhaps something that dances along the edge of quantum interaction. But it's real. It works. And it could, in principle, be studied, reverse-engineered, or replicated — assuming it hasn't already been.

What they've done to me is not magic. It's simply ahead of us.

Reflection and Speculation

I've often wondered why the trance state is so overlooked in abduction literature. Maybe it's because it doesn't lend itself to drama. There's no screaming, no struggle, no broken restraints. And yet, for me, it remains the most haunting aspect of the entire phenomenon. Not the procedures. Not the beings. Not even what was taken. But the quiet theft of self.

To be conscious without emotion, to be awake but without agency, is to exist in a kind of living suspension — not dead, not dreaming, not alive in the usual sense. And the fact that this state can be imposed externally — not as a side effect, but as part of the design — tells me more about the intelligence behind these encounters than almost anything else.

Whoever or whatever they are, they have mastered our interface. They know how to enter the mind not through words or persuasion, but through direct manipulation. They don't need to ask for compliance. They eliminate the part of us that would refuse. And in doing so, they turn a human being into something closer to a device — awake, aware, but ready to be operated.

And here's the part that stays with me: I was not afraid. I should have been. The part of me that should have protested — that primal scream of sovereignty — had been silenced with precision. That suggests something more than physical manipulation. It suggests a form of possession without force. The Greys do not need to overpower. They overwrite.

I sometimes wonder whether this trance is just a means to an end — a necessary tool to manage the subject during procedures. Or whether it's more than that. A way to study consciousness itself. To observe what happens when you isolate awareness from emotion, when you sever agency from perception. Maybe they're not just using us. Maybe they're watching what happens to us when the soul is gently pushed aside.

If so, then these encounters aren't just physical — they're experiments in consciousness. Each time they pull me inside that silent, numbed state, I become not just a subject of study, but part of a larger question: What are we, really, when all choice is removed? When the body is present, but the self has been dimmed to a whisper?

And what does it say about us — or about them — that such a state is even possible?

The trance leaves behind a strange residue. Not trauma, exactly. More like displacement. A sense that I had been inhabited, piloted, or shelved. That something had borrowed me for a while, and when it was finished, I was returned — slightly off, slightly altered. I carry that awareness now. A knowing that my body can be hijacked, my thoughts suspended, my essence filtered through someone else's lens.

It challenges everything we assume about individuality. About free will. About what it means to "be present." If someone else can access the operating system of your mind — shut down the parts that define who you are — then where, exactly, do you begin and end?

Maybe that's what they're really studying. Not just the body. Not just the mind. But the boundary between the two — and whatever flickers in between. That thing we call a soul. That thing they may not fully possess.

Maybe they don't just want to examine it. Maybe they want to know what it feels like to be inside it.

18

WHEN FAITH AND HISTORY COLLIDE

Prior to this point, I have discussed my abduction encounters and my mother's experiences dating back to the 1950's - and addressed each related topic on a broader scale, as these phenomena are widespread and generational. Over the last five years, I have had a lot of time to reflect and ponder how these experiences relate to my world view and personal beliefs. As a function of my need to understand why these incidents were occurring, and why I was chosen for what I now understand as the Greys' breeding program, I began investigating the abduction phenomenon and its history. One informational resource led to another, which brought me into the subject of "Ancient Alien Theory," whereby a wealth of historical and archaeological evidence would suggest that humanity has been interacting with - and influenced by - extraterrestrial beings for tens of thousands of years.

Now, I would like to discuss how these experiences and my research have influenced what I believe - about humanity, our origins and the religion in which I was raised. Because I am not the same. These questions didn't drive me away from belief—they changed its shape.

Yet even as these realizations unraveled the faith I was raised with, I never stopped believing in a greater intelligence. In fact, the more I learned—the more I saw the precision of nature, the structure of consciousness, the exquisite cause-and-effect in every aspect of our lives—the more convinced I became that the universe itself is the product of design. Not divine in the way the Bible taught me, but intentional. Alive with purpose.

I no longer believe in an anthropomorphic God—a bearded figure in the sky handing out blessings or punishments based on moral checklists. That idea now feels far too small. But I do believe in a creative intelligence—something vast and self-aware—that set this universe in motion with laws as elegant as gravity and as subtle as karma.

In that sense, prayer still holds value for me—not as a plea to a distant deity, but as an act of alignment. I believe the mechanism behind our reality responds to intent, emotion, and vibration. Thought, especially when focused through gratitude or longing, seems to have a directional quality. Whether we call it the Law of Attraction or something else, I've come to believe that our inner world is mirrored by the outer one—not always literally, but in deeply symbolic ways.

That realization helped me preserve a kind of faith—though it's no longer anchored to scripture. I still feel reverence. I still feel that there is more beyond this material world than we can see or measure. But I now suspect that what ancient prophets called "God" may have been something else entirely—something closer to what we now call "them."

If Abraham condensed the pantheon of the Anunnaki into a singular, all-powerful deity—if the stories of divine wrath, miracles, and chosen lineages were interpretations of extraterrestrial interaction—then our religious traditions may be the fossilized memory of a very different kind of contact. One that was never about heaven and hell, but about lineage and control.

And still, behind even the Greys and the Anunnaki, I believe something greater exists. Something that transcends biology, technology, and even time. A consciousness that births galaxies. A force that plays no favorites, but designs laws to govern balance. It's not found in commandments—it's found in cause and consequence. In what we create, and what we become.

That's where I place my faith now. Not in the gods of men, but in the intelligence behind the stars.

A Faith Once Unquestioned

I was raised in a Christian household, with faith woven into the fabric of my upbringing. My mother and father were Protestant Christians, and every Sunday morning our family attended First Congregational Church in Des Plaines, IL, part of the United Church of Christ. It was more than just a weekly obligation; it was the foundation of our values, our morals, and our understanding of the universe.

As a child, I spent every Sunday in church school, absorbing the teachings of the Old and New Testaments, just as my parents had before me. By the time I was 15 years old, I had completed my confirmation and was baptized as a follower of Christ. Christianity wasn't just a belief system I subscribed to—it was the very lens through which I understood life, death, and the meaning of existence. That lens brought comfort. I remember sitting in the pews during Sunday service, sunlight filtering through stained glass as the pipe organ filled the sanctuary with sound. The stories were ancient, but they felt close—part of a living tradition that had shaped every part of my identity. God was not just an idea; He was a presence. An anchor. A certainty. When I prayed, I believed someone was listening. When I doubted myself, I believed He had a plan.

Throughout high school and for many years after, I was deeply involved in the church. I served in the choir, singing every Sunday, filling the sanctuary with hymns that had been sung for generations before me. Even after high school, I found myself returning to the choir every holiday season for twenty years. My faith was a "given" for me. I had no reason to question the stories passed down in scripture, no reason to doubt that the events described in the Bible were divine truth. I never felt the need to compare those stories to anything else—why would I? They were self-contained, complete. There was no mention of ancient astronauts or genetic engineering in our Sunday lessons. No suggestion that the "miracles" of the Bible might have been misunderstood technologies. The idea would have sounded heretical. Unthinkable. In those years, the concept of God and the stories of scripture were inseparable—two sides of the same sacred truth.

That all began to change in 2020. It didn't happen all at once. At first, it was just discomfort—a quiet dissonance between what I was experiencing and what my faith had taught me to expect. I tried to hold on to both. I wanted the encounters to fit within the framework I'd grown up with. But they didn't. The Greys didn't speak in parables or radiate divine light. They weren't angels or demons. They were clinical, exacting, and indifferent to the rules I thought governed the spiritual world.

As I started to recall more of my abduction experiences, questions arose—questions that I couldn't ignore. I had to confront not only what was happening to me but also what it implied about the world I thought I understood. The reality of extraterrestrial contact clashed with the faith I had been raised in. I couldn't reconcile the two—not without digging deeper.

Once I began researching ancient astronaut theory, I realized that these beings had been here for a very long time—long before the birth of modern civilization. If extraterrestrials had been interacting with humanity for tens of thousands of years, how much of what we call history was influenced by their presence? How many of our religious texts were shaped by encounters that early humans could only interpret in the language of gods and miracles?

That's when I began to reexamine the stories of my faith, not as divine revelations but as possible records of contact—misunderstood and rewritten through the lens of ancient peoples. And as I studied further, it became clear to me that the roots of the Old Testament stretched far beyond Israel, beyond Moses, beyond even Abraham. They reached deep into Sumerian civilization, into texts written thousands of years before the Bible—texts that mirrored the creation and flood narratives I had once taken as truth.

How much of human history has been altered by their involvement? How many of our oldest beliefs were shaped by interactions with something not of this Earth? As I delved deeper, my perspective continued to shift, leading me to rethink the very foundation of my faith—which brings me to an important question:

What were the origins of our religious stories? And more importantly... who gave them to us?

Rewriting the Origins of Faith

For much of my life, I, like so many others, viewed the Judeo-Christian creation story as the foundation of human history. The Garden of Eden, Noah's Flood, the Tower of Babel—these were ancient stories of divine intervention, shaping the course of civilization through the will of an almighty, omnipotent God.

But as my encounters with the Greys intensified, I began to question the nature of divine intervention itself. What if God—or at least the "gods" of ancient texts—was never a single, all-powerful deity, but rather a group of advanced extraterrestrial beings who played a direct role in guiding, modifying, and selectively preserving segments of the human race?

The more I researched, the more I realized that our religious texts are not unique. The Old Testament does not exist in a vacuum—many of its most iconic stories have older, nearly identical counterparts in Sumerian mythology, dating back thousands of years before the Hebrew Bible was written.

Take Abraham, the founding patriarch of Judaism, Christianity, and Islam. He wasn't originally a Hebrew. He was a Sumerian from the great city of Ur, one of the earliest centers of human civilization. If Abraham carried his oral traditions forward when he left Sumer, then the creation story and the flood narrative would have originated not with Yahweh, but with the Sumerian gods—the Anunnaki.

To the Sumerians, the Anunnaki were the "gods" who descended from the sky, created mankind, and ruled over humanity. But to those of us who have experienced abduction, genetic harvesting, and missing time, the Anunnaki bear an eerie resemblance to the extraterrestrials described by abductees worldwide.

The Creation Myth: Enuma Elish

The creation story of Genesis bears striking similarities to the Enuma Elish, the Babylonian-Sumerian creation myth, written on seven clay tablets sometime around 1750 BCE—though the story itself is believed to be far older, tracing back to Sumerian roots.

According to the Enuma Elish, before the world existed, there was only a chaotic, primordial state, ruled by the cosmic waters Apsu and Tiamat. Over time, a new generation of gods emerged, including Enki and Marduk, who rose up against the older primordial deities. Through a process of divine conflict and creation—reminiscent of genetic manipulation described in abduction cases—Marduk ultimately defeated Tiamat, using her remains to fashion the heavens, the earth, and humanity itself.

Compare this to Genesis, where the formless void is shaped by divine command, with humanity created in the image of a supreme being. But in Sumerian accounts, humans were not created as divine children, but as servants of the gods—beings designed for labor. However, the Anunnaki did not simply create humans as mindless drones. In the Atra-Hasis, Enki and Ninhursag declare, "Let man bear the image of the gods," mirroring the Biblical phrase, "Let us make man in our image." Similarly, in the Enuma Elish, after Marduk slays Kingu, the gods proclaim, "From his blood, let us create mankind in the likeness of the gods." Yet, despite being made in their image, humans were not created to share in divine rule, but to serve—fashioned from the essence of the gods but bound to toil in their place. This aligns with theories suggesting humanity was genetically engineered by an advanced species—our purpose not to rule the world, but to serve those who created us.

The Flood Story: The Epic of Gilgamesh

The story of Noah's Ark also originates in Sumerian tradition, found in Tablet XI of the Epic of Gilgamesh—one of the oldest known written stories, dating back at least 4,000 years. But the events themselves likely date back to the late Younger Dryas period, when the ice age ended.

In this version, the Sumerian hero Ziusudra (later called Utnapishtim in the Akkadian retelling) is warned by the god Enki that a great flood is coming to wipe out humanity. He is told to build a massive boat, gather animals, and preserve life. After the flood subsides, he releases a bird to find dry land—a nearly identical sequence of events to Noah's story in Genesis.

But why did the Sumerian gods want to wipe out humanity in the first place? The texts suggest that humans had become too numerous, too noisy, and too difficult to control. If this sounds eerily familiar, it's because similar justifications have been used in modern theories of population control and hybrid integration.

Could this Great Flood have been an engineered event—an extraterrestrial attempt to reset human civilization, preserving only a small genetic sample deemed worthy of survival?

The Anunnaki's Role in Human Development

The Sumerian gods—Enki, Enlil, and the Anunnaki—were depicted not as distant, spiritual entities but as beings that walked among humans, interacted with them, and dictated the course of civilization.

Enki was the god of knowledge and creation, often seen as humanity's protector—the one who defied the others by warning Ziusudra about the flood. Enlil was the storm god, frequently portrayed as the enforcer of divine will—similar to the wrathful God of the Old Testament. The Anunnaki, whose name means "those who came from heaven to earth," were the celestial rulers who guided, manipulated, and in some cases, intervened directly in human affairs.

If Abraham carried these stories with him when he left Ur, then the books of the Old Testament are not the origin of these ideas—it is simply a later version of an older extraterrestrial narrative.

And what of Old Testament stories that came after Abraham's time? What if we view these events through the lens of Ancient Astronaut Theory? The Exodus, for instance.

The Exodus: An Engineered Migration?

If the Greys have been influencing human civilization for thousands of years, guiding certain populations while subtly manipulating history to fit their agenda, then the Exodus of the Israelites from Egypt could also be viewed in an entirely new light.

Traditionally, the Exodus story is told as a tale of divine intervention—God choosing Moses as His messenger, sending a series of plagues to break Pharaoh's will, and ultimately leading His "chosen people" to the Promised Land. But what if this event wasn't the work of an omnipotent deity in the way most believers understand, but rather the deliberate intervention of extraterrestrial beings, ensuring the preservation of a specific genetic lineage?

At the time, Egypt was a melting pot—a powerful empire that absorbed people from all over the known world, including traders, slaves, and settlers from many different backgrounds. The Israelites, living among them, were at risk of intermixing with other genetic lines, potentially diluting whatever traits the Greys were selectively curating. If the Greys had a vested interest in keeping this population as homogenous as possible, then it would make sense that they would take direct action to extract them from the diverse Egyptian landscape and isolate them elsewhere.

The Book of Exodus describes a series of plagues that forced Pharaoh to release the Israelites, each event seemingly designed to cripple Egypt's infrastructure. The first plague turned the waters of the Nile into blood, an event that could have been caused by a form of toxic algal bloom or biological contamination, possibly introduced artificially. This was followed by infestations of frogs, lice, and flies, all of which align with ecological disruptions that could have resulted from deliberate tampering with Egypt's water supply or climate. Then came diseases that struck both livestock and humans, spreading with precision as though guided by an unseen hand. If the Greys possessed advanced biological technology, these plagues could have been the result of targeted pathogens designed to weaken the Egyptian state while sparing the Israelites.

The plagues continued to escalate. Hail and fire rained down from the sky, an event that could have been the result of atmospheric manipulation or a directed energy attack. Then came the most chilling of all—the death of the firstborn sons of Egypt. This plague suggests a form of selective biological warfare, one that could target individuals based on a specific genetic marker, age, or even birth order. The fact that it affected only the firstborn, while the Israelites were seemingly untouched, raises the possibility of a highly sophisticated, genetically targeted intervention.

Once the Israelites were freed, their escape was guided by what was described as a "pillar of cloud by day and a pillar of fire by night." This imagery is eerily reminiscent of an aerial craft, leading the people through the wilderness with an advanced propulsion system that may have been beyond human understanding at the time. Then came the parting of the Red Sea, a miracle in biblical terms, but one that could also be explained through a manipulation of gravity or electromagnetic forces, temporarily displacing the waters to allow safe passage. If the Greys were capable of altering physical environments, then such an event may have been well within their technological capabilities.

This raises an even deeper question: Why did the Greys intervene at all? The Exodus was not just an escape from slavery—it was a carefully orchestrated migration event, removing a specific group from a densely populated, multi-ethnic empire and placing them into a controlled environment where their genetic purity could be maintained. Once in the wilderness, the Israelites were not simply left to their own devices. They were given a rigid set of laws and customs, including strict dietary and social regulations that discouraged intermingling with other cultures. If the Greys sought to cultivate a specific genetic line, these laws could have been a form of behavioral conditioning, ensuring the population remained isolated and did not mix with undesired genetic stock.

With this speculative framework in place, it becomes clear that the Exodus may have been one of many engineered interventions designed to shape human history. The Greys' involvement in genetic tracking, breeding programs, and hybridization efforts today may not be a recent development but the continuation of a process that has been unfolding for thousands of years. If the Israelites were guided, manipulated, and ultimately isolated for their genetic uniqueness, how many other civilizations have been influenced in similar ways throughout history? And more importantly, how many others are being influenced now?

How This Ties to My Experiences

For thousands of years, humans have believed they were being guided by divine forces. But after decades of personal experiences—abductions, telepathic communication, genetic extractions, and programmed screen memories—I began to wonder if the forces shaping human history were never truly divine at all.

Perhaps the biblical God that so many have worshiped was just one faction of an ancient extraterrestrial race, one that took an interest in a specific gene pool and sought to preserve and modify it over time.

If that's true, then the Greys today may simply be the next generation of these same beings, continuing an experiment that has been running for thousands of years.

Are we still being preserved, manipulated, and watched over, just as the ancient Sumerians described? If history is repeating itself, then humanity may be on the verge of yet another engineered transition.

If the Greys are continuing a project begun by beings once worshipped as gods, then what we've called faith may have always been, at least in part, an attempt to make sense of contact. Ancient peoples did not have a framework for technology, for genetic intervention, for mind control. What they had were stories—oral traditions passed down as myth, scripture, and eventually canon. But behind the poetry and parable may have been something far more literal: a history of manipulation disguised as divinity.

And yet, despite all I've uncovered, there's still a part of me that believes something more exists beyond these interventions—something deeper than even the Greys. I don't believe the universe is governed solely by biological engineers or data harvesters. I believe there is a soul, and I believe the soul precedes the body. I believe the laws that govern us—karma, synchronicity, the mirroring of thought and outcome—are too elegant, too finely tuned, to have been built by the Greys.

So the deeper question becomes: What are the Greys trying to reach? Why are they so focused on us—not just physically, but spiritually? What is it they see in us that they seem to lack? And what happens if they succeed in becoming part of it?

These are not just questions of science or history. These are questions of essence. Of consciousness. Of what we carry beyond the body. Of soul.

19

SOUL AGENDA

"...there is no coming to consciousness without pain."
— Carl Jung, *Metamorphosis and Symbols of the Libido*

Throughout my memoir, I have narrated for you a glimpse of what is happening to many thousands of people globally through the lens of my own experiences. It is clear to me, and to many others, that humanity is subject to an ongoing biological experiment—one in which our genetic tissues are being harvested and manipulated, splicing our race with that of another species. Or perhaps even multiple species.

Many have speculated about this breeding program, grasping at reasons to explain why the greys are creating hybrids. Are they trying to save us from our war-like ways, blending our genetics with theirs to create a kinder, more docile species? Or are they desperately trying to save themselves, a dying race incapable of natural reproduction? For nearly five years, I have wrestled with these questions, pulling from my own encounters and cross-examining them with the testimony of whistleblowers, alleged insiders, and fellow abductees. And yet, none of the prevailing theories have ever fully tracked.

Many abductees I've seen interviewed take a positive stance on the abduction phenomenon. They believe the greys are here to elevate us, to mold us into better stewards of the earth, preparing us to join some galactic community of enlightened, space-faring beings. It's a beautiful sentiment, but it's a fantasy. An illusion wrapped in comforting human projections. The truth—when you wake up to it—is not kind. As Jung said, "there is no coming to consciousness without pain." And the more I examined my own experiences, the more I came to understand that this awakening comes with a price—the destruction of naïve, human-centric assumptions. We need to exhaust all practical explanations before indulging in utopian fantasies.

Take, for example, the cattle-mutilation phenomenon. Investigators like Linda Moulton Howe have spent decades researching cattle mutilations, uncovering disturbing patterns that suggest a non-human intelligence is behind them. Some of the cases she's examined involve precision laser-like cuts, the removal of specific organs, and a complete absence of blood—hallmarks of the same kind of methodical tissue extraction that abductees have reported in their own experiences, including my own.

Livestock are abducted, drained of their blood, their organs harvested with clinical precision, and then their carcasses are discarded like bio-waste. The ease with which these animals are taken and disposed of, the total absence of concern for their suffering, is deeply telling. It suggests that the Greys do not see them as life forms deserving of compassion, but merely as resources—nothing more than convenient tissue donors. And if that is how they treat cattle, what does that imply about us?

Over time, I began to suspect that these mutilations serve at least two purposes. First, cattle may possess genetic material useful for the hybridization program. Second, and perhaps more disturbingly, their blood and tissues may be processed into a food source for the greys—a biological slurry that they absorb through their skin. Some abductees have reported that the greys they encountered had a foul, acrid odor, possibly the byproduct of excretion through their dermis. I have no memory of ever noticing such a scent, but I do recall reading purported military documents describing an autopsy of one species of grey—one that lacked a conventional digestive system entirely. If they excrete waste through their skin, it stands to reason they also absorb nutrients the same way.

The Greys treat cattle this way because they can. There is no resistance, no intervention from governments that would seek to stop them. Cattle are nothing but lab animals to them, and lab animals are not given rights. There is nothing humane in their treatment, nothing that speaks to a higher moral authority. And so I had to ask myself—why would I assume that we, as humans, are treated any differently? If the Greys were truly stewards of life, if they were acting in the best interests of planetary ecosystems, then why would their actions mirror clinical dissection rather than compassionate intervention?

And that question forced me to look at my own experiences through a new lens.

I thought about the frog-faced doctor—the one who seemed to heal my digestive tract. At first, I had assumed his presence was an act of kindness, a moment of unexpected compassion amidst a lifetime of intrusive encounters. But when I reflect on the moment again, the presence of the tall Greys in the room haunts me. They stood there, watching, observing my interaction with this being. And I began to wonder—was this about my well-being? Or was it about them?

Why would a dozen tall greys stand in quiet anticipation, breaking from whatever duties they normally perform, just to witness my interaction with a single doctor? Who am I to them?

And then it struck me. What if I wasn't just another test subject? What if I was their investment? What if every single being in that room had a personal stake in my survival?

And in that vein, I can begin to surmise their potential motivations.

The Greys' Perspective on Souls

In 1989, journalist George Knapp, working for Las Vegas' television station KLAS, broke a story of a government whistleblower who claimed to have worked at Area S4 in the Nellis Air Force Range. S4 was just fifteen miles from the infamous Area 51 where advanced aircraft are tested for the military. The whistleblower's name was eventually revealed as Bob Lazar, an engineer and physicist who admitted to being part of a back-engineering program deconstructing and reproducing captured alien spacecraft.

As part of his introduction to this back-engineering program, Lazar reported he was exposed to briefing documents that related to the aliens who supplied the technology they were studying. In one of these dossiers, it was described how the Greys of Zeta 2 Reticuli viewed human beings as 'containers.' While Lazar could only speculate on what was meant by that term, he suggested it could refer to humans being used as biological vessels, likely for genetic material. However, others in the field of abduction research have theorized that 'containers' may also refer to something far more profound—perhaps even the housing of the soul itself.

Viewing ourselves as a genetic resource to the greys may be considered somewhat "academic," or well documented at this point. What interests me, however, is the idea that we are containers of souls. What if we proceed with that assumption and try to draw some suppositions?

The tall Greys are native to a planet orbiting Zeta 2 Reticuli. This location is supported by Betty Hill's star map, the Reagan Briefing papers, Lazar's briefing dossiers and what I was told personally by Syczilick, one of the tall greys with whom I've interacted. The planet is said to be very arrid, but this would not be due to it being part of a binary star system. Zeta 1 and Zeta 2 Reticuli are far enough apart (0.06 ly) that any planet in orbit around either of them would see their companion star as merely a bright dot in the night sky. Not a second sun. It is possible, however, that over a very long time, the Greys' planet, which is purported to be smaller than earth, lost enough of its magnetic field that complex life on their planet began to sustain damage on a genetic level from solar radiation, eventually making sexual reproduction impossible for them.

Using cloning, the Greys could have engineered themselves and enough of their ecosystem to survive the radiation, but despite that were still forced to continue cloning to reproduce themselves. What if doing so affected their biology and neurology in such a way that souls could no longer be hosted within them? What if as a result of their genetic engineering, they inadvertently turned themselves into biological machines? Incapable of sexual reproduction and incapable of hosting an immortal soul?

Some people, including myself, believe that the purpose of this universe is to create and foster complex, intelligent life. We believe it is a nursery, intended to cycle a finite number of souls through organic lifespans until such time that the souls have reached a stage of development where they become viable offspring of whoever created the universe - such as a Supreme Being, or in another term, GOD. Reincarnation, therefore, would be the mechanism by which all intelligent life eventually ascends to completion.

If the Greys had bred themselves out of this "soul cycle" of development they may be seeking a way back into it.

After I came to this speculation, I began researching what other authors had to say on the subject - and this notion of Greys using hybrids to hijack our reincarnation cycles ties directly to Nigel Kerner's work in *The Song of the Greys*, where he argues that the Greys are not a natural species at all, but an artificial one, created through excessive genetic modification to the point that they severed their connection to the soul. Kerner suggests that their lack of individuality, their reliance on telepathic hive-mind communication, and their intense focus on cloning all point to one thing: they have become biological machines. And if they have lost their ability to reincarnate, then hybridization may be their only way back into the soul cycle.

Just reading this idea from another author stopped me cold in my tracks. Was our agreement pure coincidence, or have we both pieced together enough of the same clues - where only one interpretation made sense? Does our correlation equate to validation? Let's just say it encouraged me to commit the idea to this book. But it also makes me sick to my stomach.

What of Additional Authors?

Whitley Strieber, in *The Key*, describes being told by a mysterious figure that human souls retain their individuality after death, something that many other beings, including extraterrestrials, no longer possess. This echoes the findings of hypnotherapist Dolores Cannon, whose regression subjects described the Greys as being deeply involved in the process of reincarnation. Some abductees, under hypnosis, have recalled being shown souls entering bodies before birth and suggest that the Greys are trying to understand, manipulate, or even reinsert themselves into this cycle.

Dr. David Jacobs has extensively researched abduction accounts where the Greys emphasize hybrid creation, with abductees recalling the Greys showing concern for "ensuring survival"—but whose survival? If Kerner is right, the hybridization program isn't just about physical survival—it's about soul survival.

Taking Our Souls Into Perspective

Human civilization seems to rise, peak and fall in cycles. What if some of those failures were engineered to prevent us from ascending our souls to completion too quickly, thereby leaving the Greys behind in their agenda? What if the Greys used events like the Great Flood at the end of the Younger Dryas period to buy themselves enough time to genetically evolve humans to suit their needs? Humans that would be neurologically compatible enough that a tall grey's considerable intelligence and memories could be transferred into a human body that reproduces sexually and hosts a soul? In this way, Tall Greys would have a chance to reemerge into the natural cycles that permit their eventual ascension to God consciousness.

If this is the case, humanity, by cooperating with the Greys in exchange for their technology, may be selling our souls, in a manner of speaking, for trifles. Our souls would become the essence of another species, entirely, carrying their legacy into the forever after, while homo sapiens sapiens' legacy would be erased with our extinction. The beauty of our cultures would not be transferred and remembered within the realm of the creator, where we would otherwise ascend.

And what of our souls? Is this a scenario where our souls suffer as the result of no longer belonging to humanity? We ARE our souls. Our Souls are what we are. The soul is our existence. If we no longer reincarnate to human bodies, would that matter to us as souls? Would incarnating from life to life inside the bodies of Grey/Human hybrids be a bad thing?

I do not know! But this whole dynamic could be described as the Greys' usurpation of humanity's connection to immortality. Is that moot? And does our Supreme Creator Being care if our souls are from bodies that are grey, peach, brown or olive? I do not know. Should one species be able to decide for others?

A Warning From the Fields

In August of 2002, something extraordinary appeared in a wheat field near Crabwood, Hampshire, in the United Kingdom. Unlike the traditional circular and geometric crop formations that had mystified researchers for decades, this formation was different. It was complex. Deliberate. And deeply unsettling.

From the sky, it showed the unmistakable image of a Grey alien's face—constructed with precise lines and shading techniques like a halftone portrait in a newspaper. But the true enigma lay beside it: a spiral disk of intricately flattened wheat segments encoding a message in ASCII binary. Once decoded, that message delivered a chilling and cryptic warning:

"Beware the bearers of false gifts and their broken promises. Much pain but still time. There is good out there. We oppose deception. Conduit closing."

For many, this formation is nothing more than an elaborate hoax —just another entry in the long list of mysterious crop circles. But for those of us who have experienced the abduction phenomenon firsthand, the message feels eerily personal. It reads not as a metaphor, but as a transmission. A communication, likely from a faction not aligned with the Greys—or perhaps a breakaway group trying to alert humanity to what's coming.

Let's break the message down:

"Beware the bearers of false gifts and their broken promises."

This line resonates immediately with the lore surrounding the 1954 Eisenhower agreement. If the Greys offered technology in exchange for access to human subjects—and if they then exceeded those bounds—then this phrase becomes a direct indictment. A broken pact. A betrayal. The so-called "gifts" of technological knowledge may have come with strings attached—strings that bind not just governments, but human destiny itself.

"Much pain but still time."

This is perhaps the most human of the lines. It acknowledges suffering. Not just physical pain, but psychological disorientation, spiritual displacement, the quiet erosion of identity. For abductees like me, this line pierces deep. But it also carries a sliver of hope— "still time." Time for what? To resist? To awaken? To reclaim something that's being taken?

"There is good out there."

This simple sentence has profound implications. It suggests the presence of benevolent factions among the stars—perhaps those who retain their spiritual sovereignty and see what is being done to us as a violation. Maybe, like us, they have suffered under the same regimes. Maybe they evolved past it. Maybe they're trying to warn us so we don't follow the same path.

"We oppose deception."

This is where the message becomes pointed. Whoever sent it, they are directly accusing someone—likely the Greys or their collaborators—of deceiving us. Of hiding their true motives. Of leading humanity down a path that has been deliberately obscured. And this resonates with everything I've experienced: screen memories, blocked recollections, altered perceptions, and emotional numbing. Deception is the Greys' most effective tool.

"Conduit closing."

The last phrase is abrupt. It's as if the signal is cut off—or ended deliberately. The use of the word "conduit" suggests this was a transmission, a burst of information sent through an unusual channel. A temporary opportunity to speak. And then silence.

This entire formation felt like a message aimed at those who were ready to receive it—not governments, not scientists, but experiencers. People like me. People like you, the reader, who are willing to ask dangerous questions and confront uncomfortable truths.

What does it say about the phenomenon as a whole that such a message appeared in open view, yet was quickly dismissed by the media, scientists, and skeptics alike? If this truly was a communication, the failure to engage with it is another layer of the deception. The ones trying to warn us are not being heard, because the world has been conditioned to laugh at them.

But I didn't laugh. I took it seriously. Because it confirms something I've long suspected: there is a division among the non-human intelligences interacting with us. Not all are on the same team. Some may oppose what is being done. And they may not be able to interfere directly—but they can leave signs. Warnings. Messages in fields.

And what better way to bypass censorship than by flattening a message into the earth itself?

The implications are staggering. If there is a splinter group trying to warn us, then the Greys' soul agenda may be not just controversial —but unethical even by extraterrestrial standards. Perhaps there are cosmic laws we know nothing about. Laws of spiritual sovereignty. Laws that the Greys are violating.

Or perhaps it's even more personal than that. Perhaps the Greys were once part of a galactic community and were cast out because of what they became. And now, they're trying to reengineer themselves into something that passes again as "natural." Something capable of entering the reincarnation cycle, not by evolution—but by usurpation.

If that's the case, then the hybridization program is not a genetic experiment. It's a cosmic reapplication process. They are trying to forge their way back into the evolutionary ladder of spirit—using us.

And someone out there sees it. Maybe they've seen it before, on other worlds. Maybe they know how it ends.

The Crabwood message doesn't give us all the answers. It's not meant to. It's meant to wake us up. To plant a seed of suspicion in the minds of those who still believe that the Greys are saviors. That they are here to uplift us. That their gifts are anything but trojan horses.

"Beware the bearers of false gifts."

I believe we were warned. And warnings, when ignored, become regrets.

As for the Greys' attitude toward us, it could be that they consider us their "project." An ongoing development where they assume ownership and righteous mandate. As they are arguably more intelligent and advanced, they would consider their decisions and intentions as superior to our rights as a species. In a similar vein, when humans decide to build a parking lot or roadway, we give absolutely no respect to insect or rodents' nests or ant colonies that may be buried in the soil. Our needs are chosen before the needs of inferior creatures.

We are accustomed to being the superior creatures on this planet. But is that an assumption we are about to unlearn? Or will society, in general, remain in the dark until the Greys' agenda has nearly run its course? And what becomes of our species when it does? Will we gradually be phased out, as Neanderthals were by Homo sapiens sapiens? Or will humanity be culled in some disaster as engineered by the Greys?

If this is their ultimate goal—to reshape humanity into something more compatible with their needs—then the next logical question is whether our own governments are complicit in this transition. If world leaders have made deals with the Greys, whether through coercion or willing collaboration, then humanity may already be on the path toward extinction or assimilation.

Depopulation and Complicity of the Elite

If the Greys have an agenda to phase out Homo sapiens in favor of a hybrid species, the next question becomes: Are world governments complicit in this plan, or are they merely hostages to forces beyond their control?

The story begins in 1954, during the Eisenhower administration, when the United States allegedly struck a covert agreement with the Greys. According to multiple sources, President Dwight D. Eisenhower met with extraterrestrial representatives at Edwards Air Force Base, where negotiations were held in secret. In exchange for access to advanced technology, the U.S. would allow the Greys to conduct abductions for their genetic program under the condition that those taken would be returned unharmed, with no memory of the event.

At first glance, it may seem like a calculated trade—sacrificing a small number of citizens in exchange for scientific and technological leaps that could ensure military superiority. But how much control did the U.S. really have in this arrangement? Could human authorities truly enforce the terms, or was this simply an illusion of oversight, with the Greys taking whomever they pleased regardless of the agreement?

This question grows even more troubling when considering the broader global landscape. If the U.S. had entered into negotiations, what about other world powers? The Soviet Union had long been rumored to have had its own direct dealings with the Greys, with some theories suggesting that the Cold War rivalry extended beyond just human conflicts. The infamous Skinny Bob video, which appears to show a captured Grey under Soviet custody - and which I believe is authentic (despite video anamolies that sparked a debunking effort) - hints that the USSR had firsthand knowledge of these beings.

But were the Soviets partners in this exchange, or were they operating independently, seeking their own advantages? And beyond the Cold War superpowers, what role did other nations play? The British Ministry of Defence, China's military-industrial complex, and even select South American countries have long been linked to UFO secrecy, but the extent of their involvement remains unknown.

If a small, elite group of decision-makers holds the keys to these interactions, then the world's elected governments may be nothing more than puppets, managed by those who truly wield power behind the scenes. The question is whether these elites are working with the Greys willingly—or under coercion.

Engineered Population Decline – A Silent Coup?

For years, demographers have warned of a staggering decline in birthrates across the globe, a shift that has baffled scientists and policy makers alike. While mainstream explanations point to social and economic factors, a more sinister possibility emerges: Could this decline be engineered?

If a globalist elite faction is working with the Greys, then lowering the human birthrate may serve a greater purpose—one that extends far beyond traditional population control theories. A declining human population weakens civilization's ability to resist external influence, creating instability and reducing the chances of mass uprisings. But more importantly, it would pave the way for an alternative species to take root. If the Greys have long sought to introduce their own hybridized progeny, a steady drop in human reproduction would make this transition all the more seamless.

The methods of achieving such a shift remain speculative, but potential avenues exist. Some researchers have questioned whether modern medical interventions, including vaccines and pharmaceuticals, could be subtly influencing fertility over generations. Others point to chemical compounds found in food and water supplies, endocrine disruptors that alter reproductive viability in ways that are not yet fully understood. Even industrial pollutants, such as microplastics and heavy metals, could be playing a role—whether by accident or design.

If true, this suggests that the Greys would not need to force hybrid integration through open conflict. Instead, the change could unfold gradually, as natural-born hybrids increase in number while traditional human reproduction fades into the background.

Which leads to an even darker question: Are the elites doing this of their own free will, or are they being forced into compliance?

If they are willing participants, then what have they been promised in return? Have they been granted technological advancements beyond public knowledge, or the assurance of personal genetic preservation? If they are simply tools in a much larger agenda, then what happens once they have served their purpose?

The Slow Roll Toward Hybrid Integration

If the ultimate goal is the gradual replacement of Homo sapiens, then the process is already well underway—but in ways that are subtle, controlled, and strategic. There has been no sudden invasion, no global disclosure that forces humanity to confront its new reality. Instead, we are witnessing a slow and deliberate transition, where each step normalizes the next.

Cultural shifts play a role. UFO disclosure, once ridiculed, is now taken seriously at the highest levels of government, with military encounters openly discussed in congressional hearings. The scientific establishment is gradually moving toward genetic experimentation, with advancements in artificial wombs, transhumanism, and neural integration technologies—each of which could be laying the groundwork for something more profound. And at the same time, the very foundations of human civilization—economy, stability, trust in leadership—are crumbling, leaving the population vulnerable to drastic change.

If this process continues unchecked, there will come a point where humanity is no longer in control of its own fate. The question is not whether hybrids will be introduced, but whether they are already here, slowly increasing in number, waiting for the final stage of assimilation.

And when that moment arrives, what will become of the human elites who facilitated the transition? Will they still hold power, or will they simply be discarded, replaced by something else?

The true endgame remains unknown. But if the pieces are already in place, then it is only a matter of time before the next phase begins.

Reflections

As I look back on the experiences that shaped this book, one truth has become undeniable: we are not alone, and we never have been. The presence of the Greys is not a phenomenon confined to isolated abduction accounts or fragmented memories—it is a carefully executed program with a long-term strategy.

For years, I struggled to piece together the meaning behind these encounters. At first, they seemed random, chaotic—an inexplicable force disrupting my life. But with time, patterns emerged, revealing a structured and deliberate operation spanning generations. The Greys are not merely studying us; they are engineering a transition.

They have infiltrated humanity through genetic tracking, selective breeding programs, and the systematic alteration of human biology. Whether through direct abductions or through more insidious means—such as declining birthrates, hybrid integration, and the manipulation of global leaders—they are slowly reshaping the world in their image.

Their "soul agenda", if real, may be the most profound element of this entire process. The Greys' possible fascination with the human spirit, consciousness, and reincarnation suggests that their end goal is not just physical transformation but something far deeper—spiritual assimilation. If humanity's ability to reincarnate and evolve is being tampered with, then the implications extend beyond this lifetime and into the very structure of existence itself.

And then there's the question of complicity. Governments—whether willingly or through coercion—have played a role in facilitating abductions, suppressing the truth, and engineering policies that align with the Greys' objectives. The world is shifting in ways that are too coordinated to be coincidence. We see it in the collapse of societal structures, the normalization of genetic manipulation, and the slow but deliberate erosion of human autonomy.

So where does this leave us? We can choose to dismiss these realities, to look away and pretend that the changes we see are nothing more than the natural progression of society. Or we can face the truth head-on. The Greys are moving forward with their agenda whether we acknowledge it or not. The only question that remains is whether humanity will remain passive—or whether we will reclaim our fate before it is too late. But can we?

EPILOGUE

The house is quiet now. Most nights are. There's a kind of silence that settles in after midnight — not menacing, but not quite comforting either. Just present. Like something waiting for its turn. The same kind of silence that once carried shadows I didn't understand. I used to fear what might move within them. Now I simply acknowledge that they're there.

Sometimes I sit at my desk and look out into the dark, wondering if I'm being watched. Not in a paranoid way, but in the way someone wonders if they're being remembered — tagged in a system, marked for future use. The encounters have gone quiet again. But the quiet no longer feels like safety. It just feels like waiting.

This book began as an attempt to put my memories in order — to trace the arc of something I couldn't understand. But in doing that, I also ended up tracing the outline of who I've become. I don't know exactly when the shift happened, but I know I'm not the same man I was before the garage, or the orbs, or the tables. Something in me has hardened. And something else has opened. I trust less — but I perceive more.

The loss of my religious beliefs came gradually, but inevitably. The version of God I once believed in — the biblical God of Sunday mornings and quiet prayer — couldn't explain what happened to me. I don't believe in that version of God anymore. But I haven't lost faith in a higher intelligence. I still believe in a creator, or a creative force — something vast and intelligent beyond comprehension. Maybe that's what the Greys are chasing too. Or maybe they've lost it. I don't know. But I can no longer cling to stories written for a world that didn't include what I've seen.

There's no instruction manual for what happens after you go public with something like this. You can't rehearse the feeling of standing fully exposed—not because someone forced you to be, but because you finally decided it was time. Time to stop editing your memories to protect other people's comfort. Time to stop pretending the silence meant safety. Time to stop waiting for permission.

If you're reading this, it means I finally chose to speak. To break the silence. And in doing so, I crossed a line I can't uncross. For years, I was afraid to tell anyone. Not just because I feared they wouldn't believe me — but because I feared they would. That belief would open a door I could never close again.

There are still nights when I wonder if I'll be taken again. I don't know if this is over, or if it ever will be. They don't operate on a human schedule. Some of them return after weeks, others after years. For some, it's decades. If they come back for me, it might not be next month, or even next year. It could be twenty years from now, long after I've stopped looking over my shoulder. That's how they work. Time is a tool to them. And we are not the ones who hold the clock.

But I've stopped pretending. I've stopped trying to explain it away. I lived it. And if I never find out why — if no final answer ever comes — at least I've told the truth as best I could.

Sometimes I wonder what this book will become after it leaves my hands. Whether it will live in silence, tucked away on shelves or scrolled past online, or whether it will reach the kind of reader who has also woken up in places they couldn't explain. I didn't write this for fame, or validation, or even vindication. I wrote it for the one person who's still too afraid to speak. The one whose memories don't make sense—but whose instincts say they're real.

If that's you, then know this: you're not imagining it. You're not broken. You're not alone.

We don't always get answers. We don't always get justice. But we do get choices. We get to decide what we carry—and what we lay down. I've carried this burden in silence for most of my life. Now I've laid it down, page by page, word by word. That doesn't mean the weight is gone. It means I've learned how to walk with it. And if you've been carrying something too—something heavy and unspeakable—I hope this book gives you permission to set it down for a while. Or to share it. Or to name it out loud for the first time.

Because the truth is, the real transformation didn't happen during the encounters. It happened here—in the telling. That's when I began to change. That's when I reclaimed my own narrative. And that's where healing begins.

There's a kind of clarity that comes after enough silence. You stop needing it to make sense. You just carry it — not as a wound, but as a weight with which you've learned to walk.

The angst is still there, but it no longer owns me. It used to live in the shadows — in closets, in memory gaps, in the long nights between visits. Now, I face it with open eyes. I've made peace with the shadows. And maybe that was the point all along. Not to banish the angst …but to walk through it. And I have.

If they return, I'll be ready—not with fear, but with clarity. I don't need to understand everything to stand my ground. I've made peace with the questions. And if this journey continues beyond these pages, I'll meet it with open eyes. Because now, the shadows no longer chase me.

SOURCES & FURTHER READING

The following books, studies, and declassified documents provide further insight into the topics discussed in this memoir. These sources explore the abduction phenomenon, alien implants, hybridization programs, government-ET agreements, and globalist involvement in potential depopulation efforts. Additionally, they examine historical records, ancient texts, and theories on extraterrestrial influence, genetic manipulation, and the possible role of the Greys in shaping human spirituality and reincarnation.

I did not discover these sources all at once. They emerged slowly, like mile markers on a journey I never intended to take—but once I started down the path, I couldn't turn away. Some of these books gave me language for things I had experienced but couldn't explain. Others challenged my assumptions, broadened my scope, or simply reminded me that I wasn't the first to ask these questions.

If you've come this far, you may be searching too. My dearest hope is that these works will serve you the way they served me—as a compass in the dark.

> "Live the questions now. Perhaps then, someday far in the future, you will gradually, without even noticing it, live your way into the answer."
> — Rainer Maria Rilke, *Letters to a Young Poet*

Abduction & Implant Phenomenon

1. **Strieber, Whitley** – *Communion: A True Story.* New York: Morrow, 1987.

2. **Strieber, Whitley** – *The Key: A True Encounter.* 2011.

3. **Leir, Roger** – *The Aliens and the Scalpel: Scientific Proof of Extraterrestrial Implants in Humans.* Book Tree, 1999

4. **Sims, Derrel** – *Alien Hunter: Evidence and Truth About Alien Implants.* 2014.

5. **Hopkins, Budd** – *Intruders: The Incredible Visitations at Copley Woods.* 1987.

6. **Jacobs, David M.** – *The Threat: The Secret Agenda: What the Aliens Really Want... and How They Plan to Get It.* 1998.

7. **Jacobs, David M.** – *Walking Among Us: The Alien Plan to Control Humanity.* 2015.

8. **Dennett, Preston** – *The Healing Power of UFOs: 300 True Accounts of People Healed by Extraterrestrials.* Blue Giant Books, 2018.

- A comprehensive catalog of cases involving physical and emotional healing following contact with UFOs, orbs, and alien beings. Includes detailed accounts of hospital-room visitations, terminal illness remission, and unexpected recoveries documented by experiencers and witnesses.

Government-ET Agreements & UFO Secrecy

9. **Good, Timothy** – *Above Top Secret: The Worldwide UFO Cover-Up.* 1987.

10. **Good, Timothy** – *Need to Know: UFOs, the Military, and Intelligence*. 2007.

11. **Corso, Philip J.** – *The Day After Roswell*. 1997.

12. **Dolan, Richard** – *UFOs and the National Security State*. 2002.

13. **Dolan, Richard M.** – *The Alien Agendas: A Speculative Analysis of Those Visiting Earth*. 2020.

14. **Salla, Michael E.** – *Exopolitics: Political Implications of the Extraterrestrial Presence*. 2004.

15. **Jacobsen, Annie** – *Area 51: An Uncensored History of America's Top Secret Military Base*. 2011.

16. **Howe, Linda Moulton** – *Glimpses of Other Realities: Vol. I & II*. 1993, 1998.

Globalist Agendas & Population Control

17. **Engdahl, F. William** – *Seeds of Destruction: The Hidden Agenda of Genetic Manipulation*. 2007.

18. **Jones, Alex** – *The Great Reset: And the War for the World*. 2022.

19. **Coleman, John** – *The Committee of 300*. 1991.

20. **Marrs, Jim** – *Rule by Secrecy*. 2000.

Declassified Government Documents & Leaked Reports

21. **Majestic 12 (MJ-12) Documents** – Alleged classified documents detailing U.S. government knowledge of extraterrestrial beings and agreements.

22. **CIA UFO Documents (2021 Release)** – Declassified government reports on UFO encounters, secrecy, and national security implications.

23. **RAND Corporation 1968 UFO Study** – A government-funded analysis of UFOs and their possible impact on global security.

24. **Project Serpo Documents** – Alleged classified reports detailing a U.S. exchange program with Greys, involving human personnel traveling to an extraterrestrial planet.

Ancient Sumerian Texts & Sources on Early Mythology

25. **The Enuma Elish** – The Babylonian Epic of Creation
    - While Babylonian in origin, this text shares deep ties to Sumerian creation myths and influenced later Abrahamic traditions.

26. **The Atrahasis Epic** – The Babylonian Flood Story
    - A significant predecessor to the Noahic flood myth, describing the creation of mankind by the gods and their eventual near-destruction.

27. **The Eridu Genesis** – The Sumerian Creation & Flood Narrative
    - The oldest known account of the Great Flood, divine intervention, and human preservation—elements that later appear in Genesis.

28. **The Sumerian King List** – A Record of Kingship "Descending from Heaven"
    - A mix of mythology and history, this document claims kingship was granted to humans by the gods, with rulers living for impossibly long lifespans—echoing biblical patriarchs.

29. **The Epic of Gilgamesh** – The First Heroic Quest & Flood Connection
    - One of the oldest recorded epics, featuring a divine-human hybrid hero, a search for immortality, and a flood story parallel to Noah's Ark.

Scholarly & Analytical Works on Ancient Myth & Religion

30. **Kramer, Samuel Noah** – *History Begins at Sumer: Thirty-Nine Firsts in Recorded History* (1956)
    - A foundational text by one of the leading Sumerologists, detailing how Sumerian civilization shaped modern religious and societal concepts.

31. **Kramer, Samuel Noah** – *The Sumerians: Their History, Culture, and Character* (1963)

- A detailed exploration of Sumerian culture, including their pantheon of gods, early science, and influence on later civilizations.

32. **Dalley, Stephanie** – *Myths from Mesopotamia: Creation, The Flood, Gilgamesh, and Others* (1991)
- A comprehensive translation of key Mesopotamian myths, including Enuma Elish, Atrahasis, and Gilgamesh, with commentary on their biblical parallels.

33. **Sitchin, Zecharia** – *The 12th Planet* (1976)
- A controversial but widely read interpretation of Sumerian myths, proposing an ancient astronaut theory centered around the Anunnaki.

34. **Collins, Andrew** – *The Gods of Eden: Egypt's Lost Legacy and the Genesis of Civilization* (2002)
- While focused on Egypt, Collins explores Sumerian connections to biblical stories and extraterrestrial influence on early civilizations.

Soul Manipulation & Hybridization

35. **Kerner, Nigel** – *The Song of the Greys: UFOs and the Destiny of Mankind* (1997)
- A deeply researched theory that the Greys are artificial biological entities created through genetic modification, severing their connection to the soul.

36. **Kerner, Nigel** – *Grey Aliens and the Harvesting of Souls: The Conspiracy to Genetically Tamper with Humanity* (2010)
- Explores the idea that the Greys' hybridization program is not merely biological, but a desperate attempt to regain access to the reincarnation cycle.

37. **Cannon, Dolores** – *The Custodians: Beyond Abduction* (1998)
- Based on hypnotic regressions, this book suggests the Greys are deeply involved in monitoring and influencing human reincarnation.

38. **Cannon, Dolores** – *Keepers of the Garden* (1993)
- A regression-based study that explores claims of extraterres-

trials overseeing Earth's spiritual development and reincarnation cycles.

Subterranean Alien Bases & Hidden Civilizations

39. **Goodman, Jeffrey** – *American Genesis: The American Indian and the Origins of Modern Man* (1981)
- Explores Native American myths, including the Hopi legends of the Ant People and their underground refuge during global cataclysms.

40. **Lloyd, Harold T. Wilkins** – *Mysteries of Ancient South America* (1945)
- Investigates theories that ancient subterranean cities existed in South America, linked to pre-Columbian myths of underground gods.

41. **MacRae, Stuart** – *The Hollow Earth Enigma* (1979)
- Discusses early Hollow Earth theories and their relationship to legends of hidden subterranean civilizations.

42. **Heiser, Michael S.** – *The Facade* (2007)
- A well-researched blend of biblical analysis and ancient astronaut theory, including Agartha, Shambhala, and the Book of Enoch's accounts of underground realms.

43. **Sitchin, Zecharia** – *The Stairway to Heaven* (1980)
- Examines the Anunnaki's underground "Abzu" domain, where early humans were allegedly genetically engineered.

Modern UFOlogy & Underground Alien Bases

44. **Schneider, Phil** – *The Underground Alien Bases of Dulce, New Mexico* (1996)
- Explores first-hand accounts of Dulce Base, whistleblower testimonies, and alleged hybrid experimentation.

45. **Lazar, Bob** – *Dreamland: An Autobiography* (2019)
- Bob Lazar's first-hand account of working at Area S4, including briefings about underground ET facilities and transport systems.

45. **Redfern, Nick** – *Bloodline of the Gods: Unraveling the Mystery of the Human Blood Type to Reveal the Aliens Among Us* (2015)
- Examines government knowledge of genetic tampering, hybrids, and underground alien influence.

47. **Warren, Michael & Steiger, Brad** – *Underground Alien Bases* (2013)
- A deep dive into underground UFO bases, including Dulce, Mount Shasta, and global subterranean networks.

48. **Leir, Roger** – *Casebook: Alien Implants* (1999)
- Discusses possible implant tracking of abductees and underground breeding facilities.

49. **Dolan, Richard** – *UFOs and the National Security State*, Vol 2 (2009)
- Covers classified government knowledge of underground alien operations and the military's involvement.

50. **Hamilton, Norio** – *Dulce Base: The Truth and Evidence from the Case Files of Gabe Valdez* (2018)
- One of the most detailed investigations into Dulce Base and its connections to hybrid experimentation.

Ancient Underground Structures & Advanced Engineering

51. **Childress, David Hatcher** – *Lost Cities & Ancient Mysteries of the Southwest* (1989)
- Investigates ancient subterranean tunnels, Hopi lore, and deep cave systems linked to ET theories.

52. **Childress, David Hatcher** – *Lost Cities of China, Central Asia, and India* (1991)
- Covers Shambhala, Agartha, and lost underground cities rumored to house extraterrestrial beings.

53. **Tellinger, Michael** – *Slave Species of the Gods: The Secret History of the Anunnaki and Their Mission on Earth* (2005)
- Discusses the Anunnaki's genetic modifications of humans and their hidden underground bases.

54. Emery, Clifford & Fossett, Ron – *Secret Underground Bases and Facilities* (2011)
- Details government and private-sector subterranean facilities used for classified ET projects.

Additional Government & Declassified UFO Documents

55. Project Serpo Documents – Alleged classified U.S. government reports detailing human-extraterrestrial exchange programs with underground bases.

56. RAND Corporation 1968 UFO Study – A government-funded analysis of UFO secrecy and potential underground installations.

57. Majestic 12 (MJ-12) Documents – Alleged reports outlining government-ET agreements and hybridization programs.

58. The Reagan Briefing Papers – Allegedly declassified memos discussing Zeta Reticuli, genetic experiments, and the Grey agenda.

Abduction Patterns & Long-Term Monitoring

59. Sparks, Jim – *The Keepers: An Alien Message for the Human Race* (2006)
- A firsthand abductee account describing structured visitation schedules, long-term abduction cycles, and telepathic communications with non-human entities.

60. Lamb, Barbara – *Alien Experiences: 25 Cases of Close Encounter* (2008)
- A case study collection from hypnotherapy sessions, documenting abductees who were taken in 20+ year intervals and those who experienced multi-generational abductions.

Stem Cell Research & Genetic Monitoring

61. Goodell, Margaret A., et al. – "*Hematopoietic Stem Cell Plasticity: Time for a Re-Evaluation?*" (2015) Nature Reviews Molecular Cell Biology

- Discusses the regenerative potential of bone marrow stem cells, their ability to produce diverse cell types, and their role in long-term biological research.

62. **Trounson, Alan & McDonald, Claire** – *"Stem Cell Therapies in Clinical Trials: Progress and Challenges"* (2015) Cell Stem Cell Journal
- Explores the long-term applications of stem cells in medicine, hinting at why the Greys may continue taking biological samples beyond reproductive viability.

Neural Plasticity & Cognitive Tracking

63. **Pascual-Leone, Alvaro, et al.** – *"Neuroplasticity: Changes in Gray and White Matter Structure in Response to Learning and Experience"* (2005) Annual Review of Neuroscience
- A study demonstrating how the brain continually rewires itself across the human lifespan, which could explain why the Greys repeatedly monitor abductees' neurological development.

Epigenetics & Multi-Generational DNA Monitoring

64. **Jaenisch, Rudolf & Bird, Adrian** – *"Epigenetic Regulation of Gene Expression: How the Environment Can Shape Inheritance"* (2003) Nature Reviews Genetics
- Explores how epigenetic markers change over a person's lifetime, influencing genetic expression in offspring—a concept highly relevant to multi-generational abductions.

65. **Jirtle, Randy L. & Skinner, Michael K.** – *"Environmental Epigenomics and Disease Susceptibility"* (2007) Nature Reviews Genetics
- Details how environmental and external influences can alter genetic expression without changing the underlying DNA sequence, raising the question of whether abductees' DNA is being actively manipulated over generations.

Mind Control, Hypnosis & Consciousness Studies

66. Hufford, David J. – *The Terror That Comes in the Night: An Experience-Centered Study of Supernatural Assault Traditions.* University of Pennsylvania Press, 1982.

- A groundbreaking anthropological and phenomenological study of sleep paralysis, out-of-body states, and perceived entity encounters, with direct parallels to abduction cases.

67. Spiegel, David – *"Hypnosis Modulates the Default Mode Network."* Nature Communications, 2016.

- fMRI-based study showing that hypnotic trance reduces executive brain activity and alters self-awareness — supporting parallels with the entranced state reported by abductees.

68. Erickson, Milton H. – *Collected Papers on Hypnosis.* Various publications, 1950s–1970s.

- Seminal writings from the founder of modern hypnotherapy, describing trance as a shift in brain state with specific physiological markers.

69. Weihrer, Carol – *Testimony on anesthesia awareness before U.S. Congress,* 2000.

- A rare firsthand account of conscious paralysis during surgery, used widely in patient rights advocacy and medical ethics reform.

70. Ghoneim, Mohamed M. & Block, Richard I. – *"Learning and Memory During General Anesthesia: An Update."* Anesthesiology, vol. 87, no. 2, 1997.

- An influential paper exploring how some patients under general anesthesia retain partial awareness — a medical parallel to abduction trance states.

71. Van der Kolk, Bessel – *The Body Keeps the Score: Brain, Mind, and Body in the Healing of Trauma.* Viking, 2014.

- Foundational work on how trauma is stored in the body and brain, including dissociative states and emotional silencing.

72. Simeon, Daphne & Abugel, Jeffrey – *Feeling Unreal: Depersonalization Disorder and the Loss of the Self.* Oxford University Press, 2006.

- Examines the experience of feeling disconnected from one's body or emotions — relevant to the clinical side of abduction-induced entrancement.

PHOTO GALLERY

These images are visual reconstructions—composites built from memory, emotion, and careful reflection. Some depict the rooms and moments I witnessed firsthand. Others are symbolic representations of experiences I struggled to describe in words alone. They are not meant to prove anything, only to invite you deeper into the story... into the shadows I once walked through alone.

I believe that illustrations are a powerful way to communicate memories and make experiences more relatable. It is my fervent hope that sharing these will resonate with other experiencers and with those who are eager to learn more about this phenomenon.

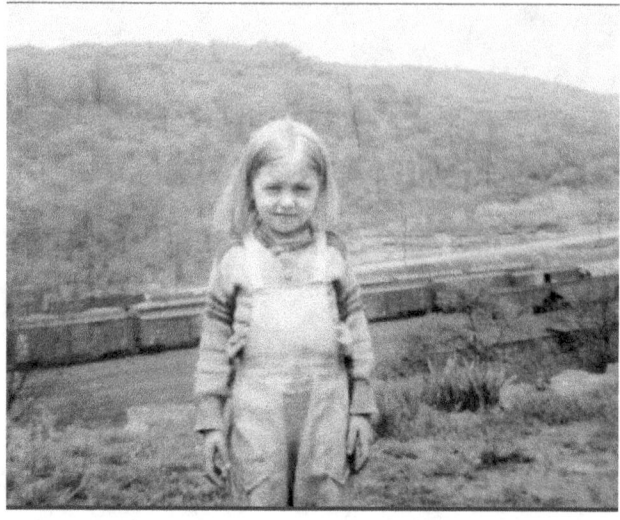

1950, Turtle Creek, Pennsylvania.

Spring 1950

Betty Jackson (Nanstiel), the author's mother as she appeared a few years prior to her suspected 1953 abduction encounter, following a UFO sighting above her childhood home.

PHOTO GALLERY

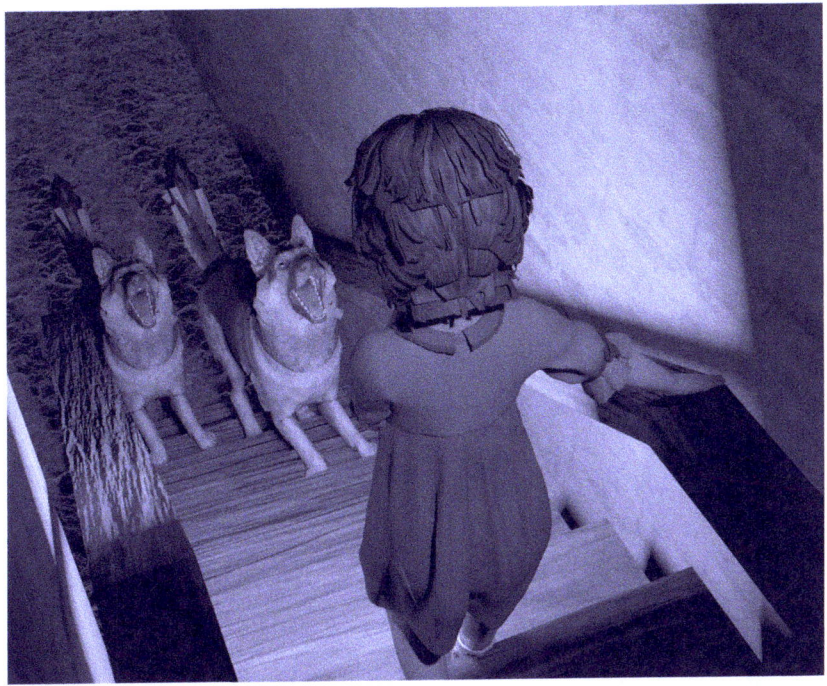

Summer 1953, Turtle Creek, PA.

Summer 1953

The author's mother, Betty Jackson (Nanstiel) awakes in the middle of the night, just hours after her brothers witnessed a UFO in the sky above their home. Compelled to descend into the basement, she encounters two angry German shepherds before blacking out - a likely screen memory consistent with many reported abduction accounts.

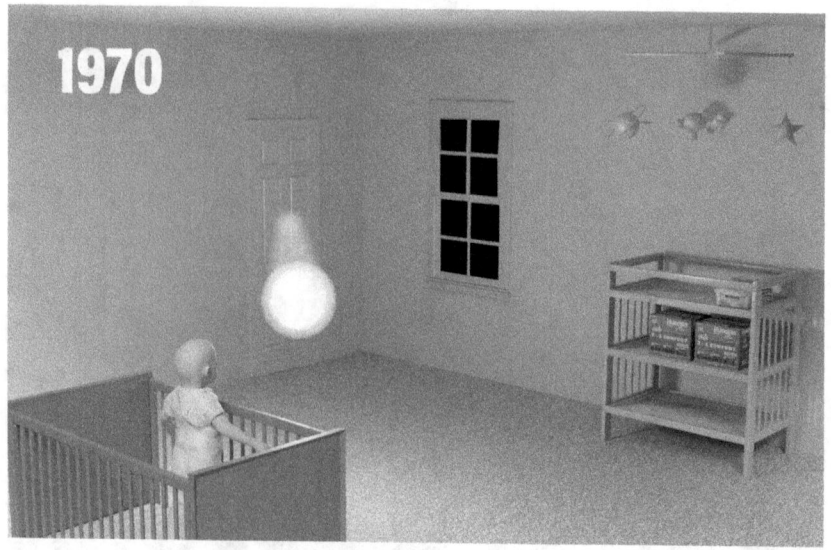

Spring 1970 Des Plaines, IL

Spring 1970

The author encounters a white, glowing orb of plasma that enters the room through his closet door and makes contact with his forehead, rendering him unconscious. This will be a recurring experience for the next four years.

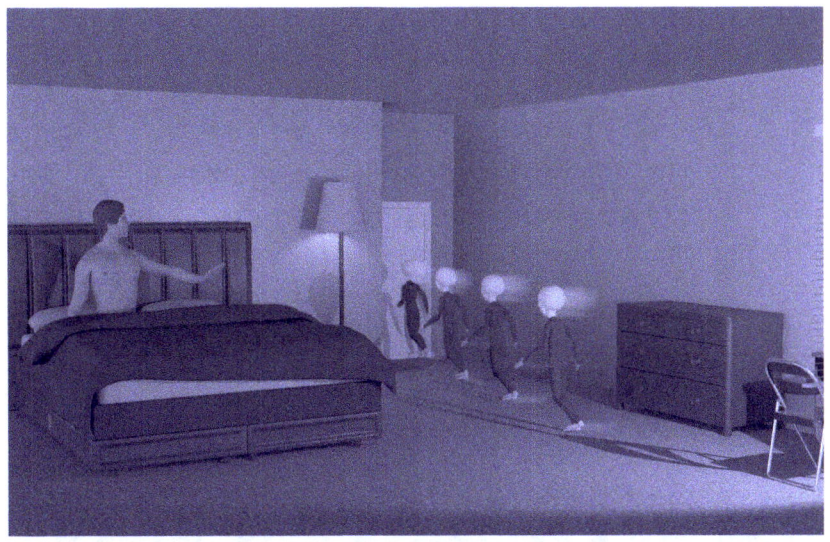

August 20, 1994 Wheeling, IL

August 20, 1994

On Saturday, August 20, 1994, the author awakens suddenly to discover four small greys rushing out of his room, passing through his bedroom door with no impediment.

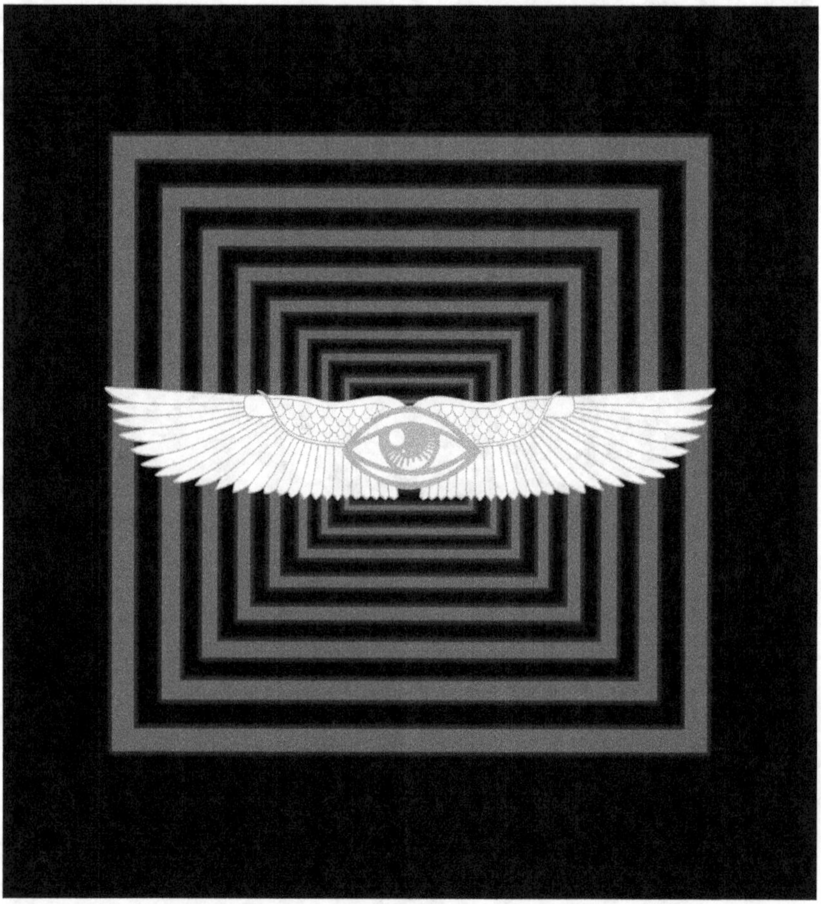

1995, Wheeling, IL

1995: A Great Eye with Wings

In a lucid dream, the author is shown a vision in response to a subconscious question: A great eye with feathered wings, backed by a series of concentric squares that pulsed in brightness in the brightest, living magenta. The author later learned that this symbol was first used in ancient Sumer - and later, Egypt.

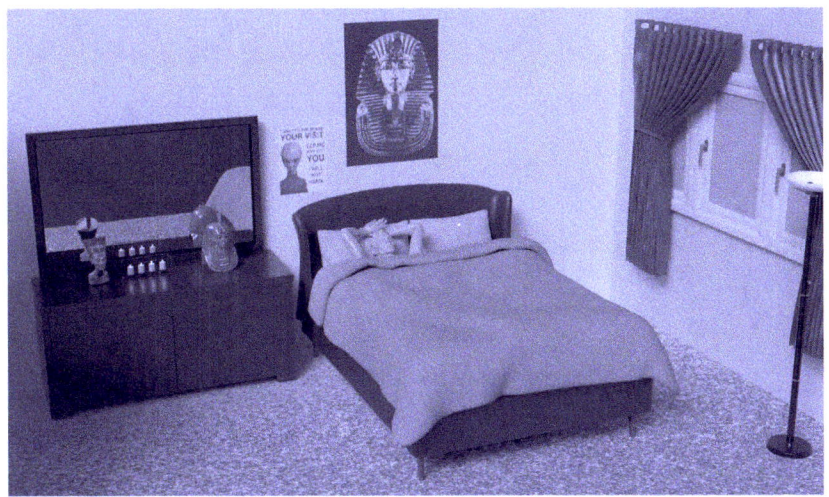

April 2020: The Wall Poster.

April 2020: The Wall Poster

This diorama accurately depicts the layout of my bedroom in 2020. Above my bed is the sign I used to communicate with whoever was entering my room while I slept - disturbing or displacing items that caught my attention the next morning.

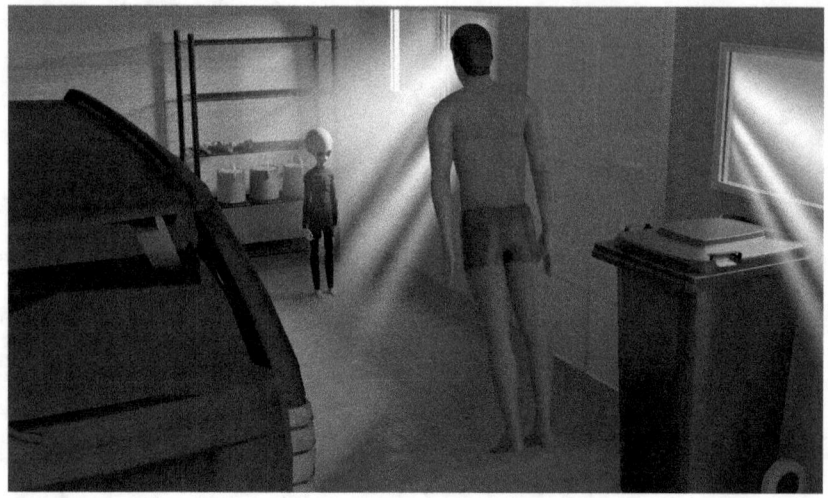

April 2020, Hoffman Estates, IL

April 2020: Garage Encounter

Depicted here is the author's garage encounter, which occurred in response to the poster he placed above his bed. The small grey communicated telepathically, saying "We can not allow you to remember our visit, or my superiors will know about it."

PHOTO GALLERY

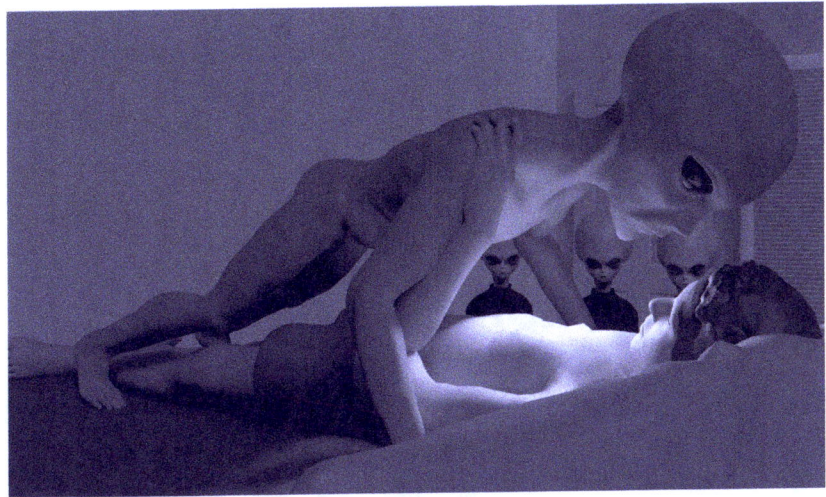

April 2020, Hoffman Estates, IL

April 2020: Bedroom Encounter with a Tall Grey

The author awakens one week after his garage encounter to discover a "tall" grey hovering on top of him. In this incident, the author touched the grey's shoulder before being rendered unconscious and into an induced REM sleep where the two communicated. Three small greys were adjacent to the bed, watching the exchange.

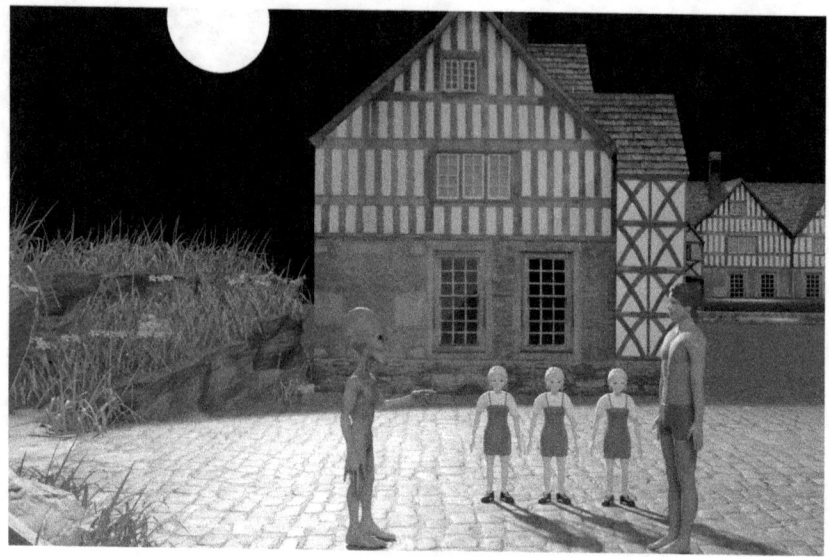

April 2020, Hoffman Estates, IL

April 2020: "Syczilick" Communicates via Induced Dream State

During the bedroom encounter with a tall grey, the author is put into an induced dream state where he is able to telepathically communicate with the tall grey and three small greys who accompanied him, but appeared as young, identical girls. The environment resembled a Bavarian village. The author learns the tall grey is named "Syczilick."

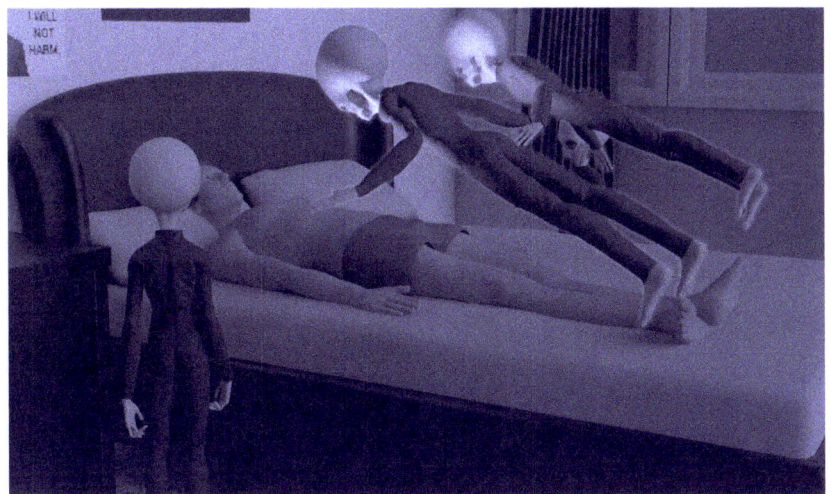

June 2020, Hoffman Estates, IL

June 2020: Two Greys Levitate over the Author's Bed

In June of 2020, the author awakens and struggles to remain conscious as he witnesses four small greys in his room. Two of the greys trade positions around the bed by levitating above the bed.

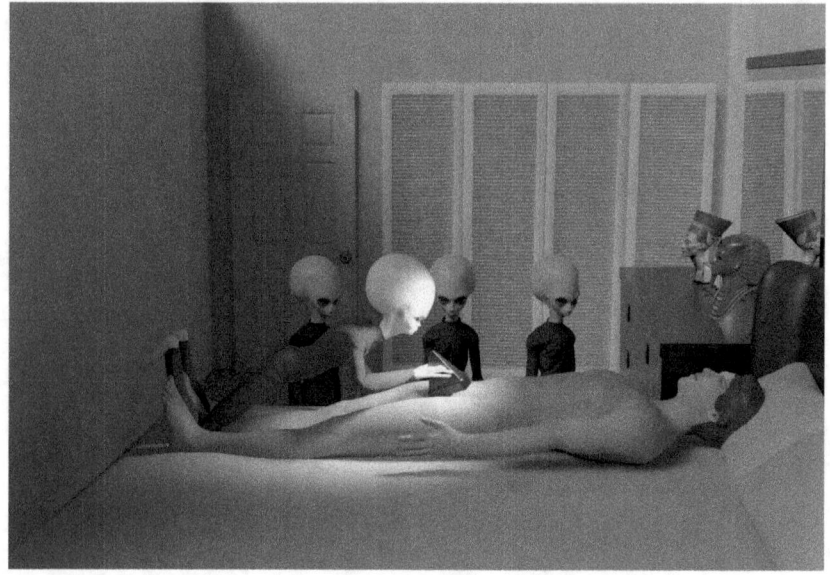

July 2020: Hoffman Estates, IL

July 2020: Four Greys Extract Semen Sample

During a July, 2020 visit, the author awakens to discover four greys engaged in a semen extraction. A black, triangular cone device is used to take the sample.

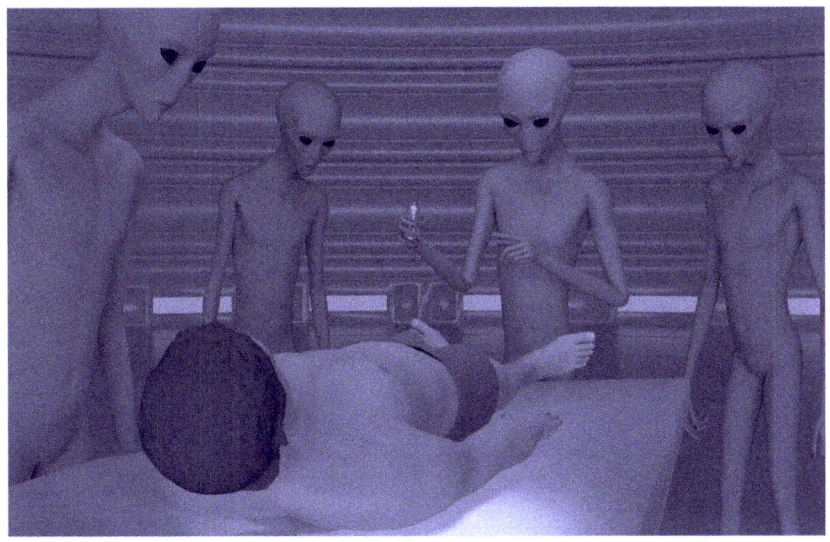

March 2021, Location Unknown

March 2021: Four Tall Greys Implant a Device into the Author's Abdomen.

The author awakens to find that he is not at home, but in a strange room, surrounded by four tall greys. One of the greys holds up a device and indicates that they are giving him a new implant that will track his location.

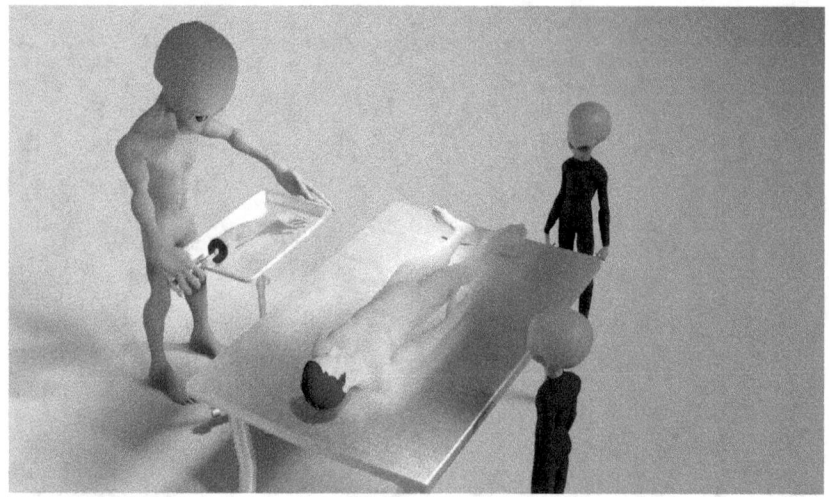

July 2022: Location Unknown

July 2022: The Surgery

The author awakens in a room with grey walls, lying on a grey metal table. In great pain, he witnesses his surgically-severed left arm laying on a metal cart beside his table.

PHOTO GALLERY

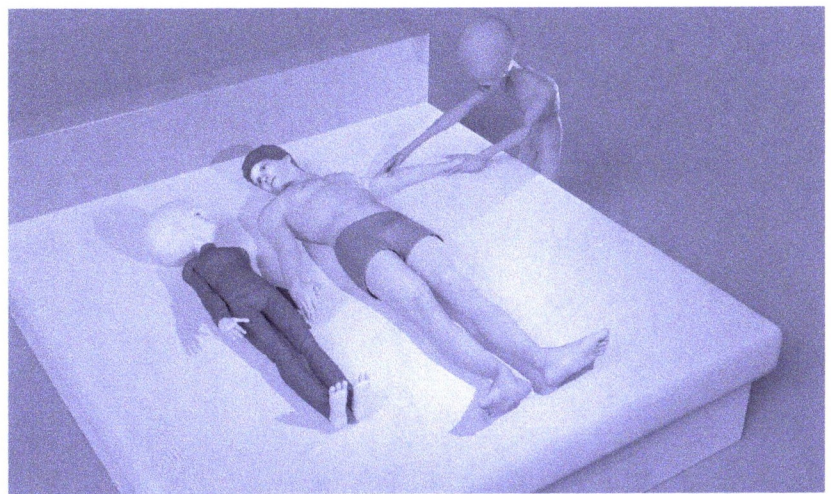

July 2022, Location Unknown

July 2022: The Surgery Follow-Up

A week after the author's arm was surgically removed and reattached, he awakens to find himself on a cushioned, white bed. A tall grey inspects his left arm while a small grey holds his right hand and asks him a question.

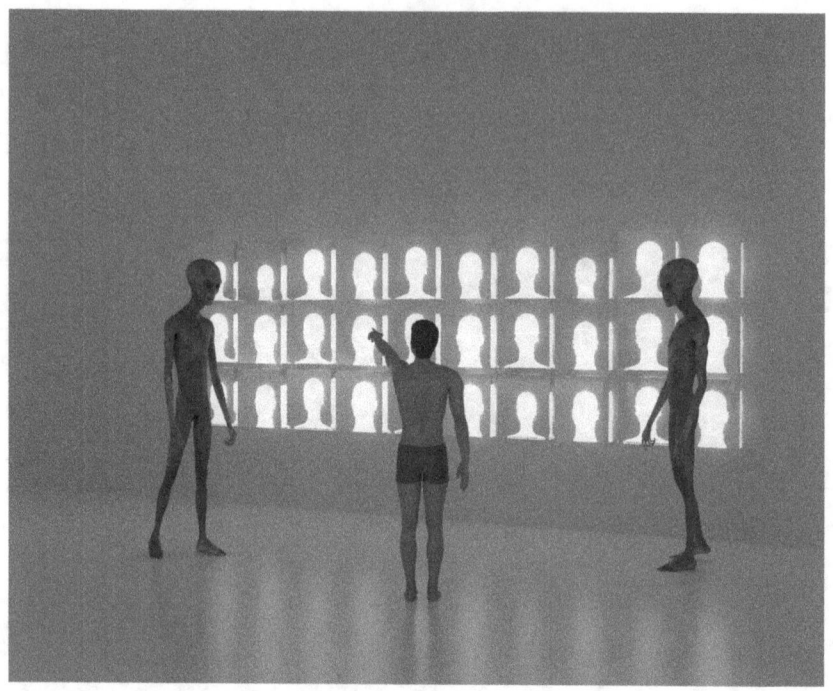

September 2022, Location Unknown

September 2022: The Children on the Wall

The author awakens in a standing position, and is confronted by two tall greys who show him a wall screen that projected portraits of his many hybridized offspring. The author is invited to name his offspring.

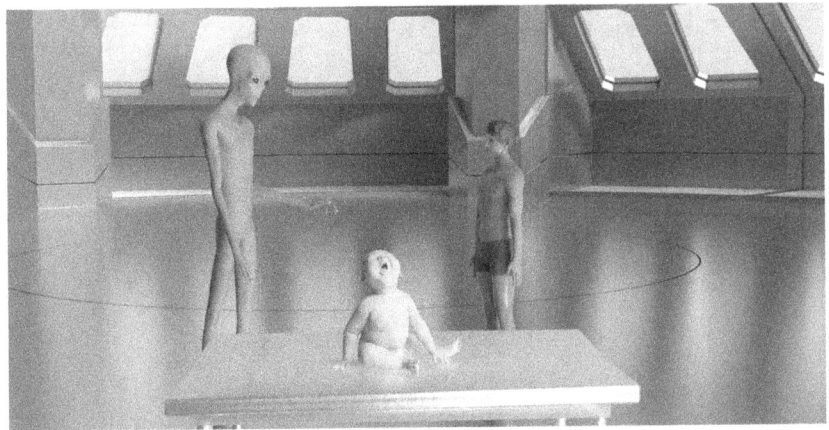

June 2023: Location Unknown

June 2023: The Baby Presentation

The author awakens in a large-diameter round room, encircled by narrow windows. Accompanying him is a tall grey who presents him with a six-month old baby boy crawling on a table in the center of the room. The child is presented as one of the author's offspring.

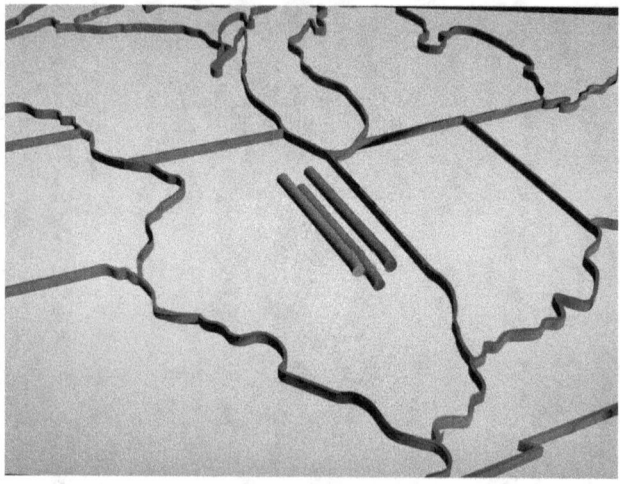

July 2023: Eastern Illinois

July 2023: The Map

The author awakens in a standing position inside a grey room, surrounded by four tall greys. When asked where the author's hybridized offspring are kept, the greys show him a 3-dimensional map depicting the location of 3 massive caverns beneath eastern Illinois.

This illustration, while not fully accurate to scale, is visually very similar to the monochrome map the author was shown.

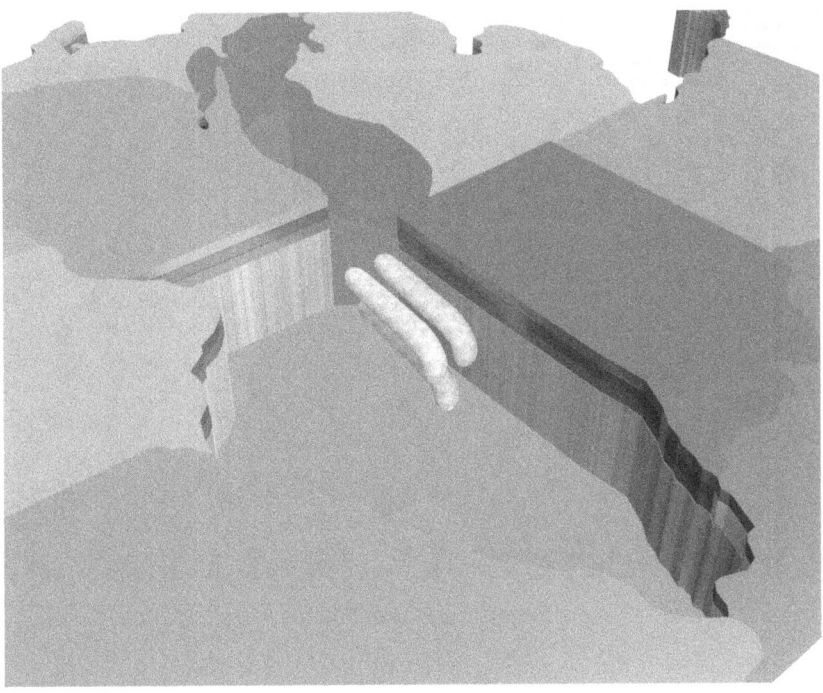

July 2023: The Map (enhanced illustration)

Depicted is a color-enhanced, more accurate-to-scale map depicting the caverns revealed to the author as the location of his hybridized offspring - in Eastern Illinois. The caverns exist at a depth of one third to one half mile.

∾

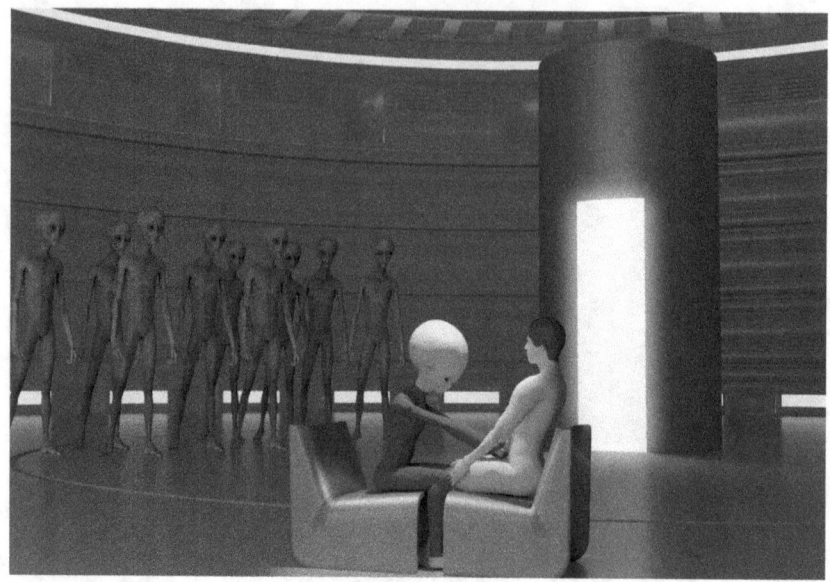

August 2023, Location Unknown

August 2023: The Doctor Will Touch You Now

The author awakens in a strange, dimly-lit room and finds he is being examined by a "doctor" who heals his gastrointestinal disorder. Looking onward from the back of the room are more than a dozen tall greys.

www.ingramcontent.com/pod-product-compliance
Lightning Source LLC
Chambersburg PA
CBHW050524100526
44581CB00006B/124/J